MW00473830

chilDREN AT bIRTh

by
THE HATHAWAYS
Jay & Marjie
Odell, Susan, Constance
James, Bobby & Ann

Photographs by
JAY HATHAWAY
and many others

Foreword by
ROBERT A. BRADLEY, M.D.
President, American Academy of
Husband-Coached Childbirth

Library of Congress Catalog Number 78-53647

ISBN Number 0-931560-00-4

Published by:
ACADEMY PUBLICATIONS
Box 5224
Sherman Oaks, CA 91413

tHE bRAdlEy METHod ®

®

AMERicAN AcAdEMy
of
husbANd-coAcHEd
childbiRTH

The American Academy of Husband-Coached Childbirth was founded by Robert Bradley,
M.D., and Jay and Marjie Hathaway for the purpose of making childbirth education information available. The Academy provides Communications Services, Resource Information, Film Showings, Lectures, Workshops, and National Affiliation for teachers.

For the protection of the public, the terms "The Bradley Method" and "Husband-Coached
Childbirth" have been registered. Only those teachers currently affiliated with the
Academy may teach the Bradley method.

"IT'S NOT NICE TO FOOL MOTHER NATURE"

Robert A. Bradley, M.D.

"THERE IS A CHILD PRESENT AT EVERY BIRTH"

Bob Kinsella, AAHCC

TO THE TRUSTING, VULNERABLE UNBORN

WHO NEED THEIR FAMILY TO BE

FETAL ADVOCATES

M & J

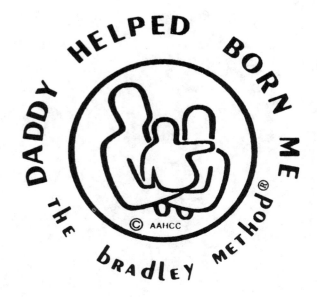

DADDY HELPED BORN ME
THE bradley METHOD®
© AAHCC

TABLE OF CONTENTS

HAVING A BABY IS AN EXPERIENCE

*which should be
well rooted
in love*

*supported by a
strong husband*

*sustaining
a wife*

*who
flowers
beautifully
in. . .*

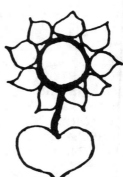

Marjie's Flower

"CHILDBIRTH FOR THE JOY OF IT"

FOREWORD

ON CHILDREN OBSERVING HUMAN BIRTHS

My lifetime interest in obstetrics began very early in my career as a farm boy on a small Kansas farm. We had horses, cows, goats, sheep, dogs and innumerable cats on our farm.

One of the most pleasant, happy aspects of my childhood was to observe the wonderful creation of new life when our animals gave birth to their young. We farm

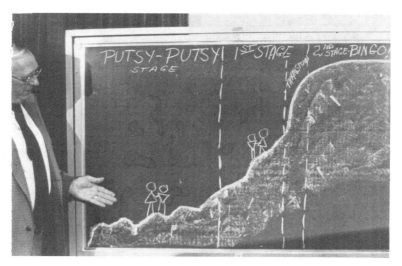

From the film, "Bradley on Birthing."

children shared the exuberance of the animal mothers and took delight with them in the cute antics of their newborn. Babies are babies, regardless of species, and are all so lovable in their helpless innocence and awkwardness.

The happy shiny-eyed mothers so freely giving of their tender mother-love to their newborns was recalled many years later when I went to medical school and observed with revulsion and horror the routine "knock-'em-out" "drag-'em-out" use of drugs and "deliveries" of human babies. From this wide contrast came my theory 31 years ago of natural childbirth for humans as described in my book, "Husband-Coached Childbirth."

Can non-instinctual human beings be taught to conduct themselves similar to other pregnant instinctual mammals and give birth to their young, joyfully and happily? Indeed they can and from such similar joy and happiness as manifested by the animals' births and trained human natural births, I was the first doctor to invite the father of the baby to be present in the "delivery room" and share in the joy of the mother.

This was the first step in my determination to make maternity hospitals home-like, the inclusion of the father of the baby. All hell broke loose in opposition by my peers in medicine and by eagle-eyed matron O.B. supervisors (nearly all old maids!) who didn't want that "dirty" husband contaminating their "sterile" delivery rooms.

Thirty-one years have gone by but my ideas of husband-coached childbirth are now nearly universally accepted internationally. Not by virtue of my medical peers but by virtue of consumer pressure, of determined young parents who refused to walk in the outmoded pathways of ancient medical ritual. Doctors are followers, not leaders, and well they should be for aren't we really public servants?

But the war is not over yet even though one battle has been won. I also observed, after being chastised by my farmer father, that we kids must not immediately take the babies away from the animal mothers to play with them for upon trying to return them to the mother later, the mother would act most un-motherly and even totaly reject the baby, even kill it.

In human comparison we are striving today to keep human, natural childbirth babies with mothers, rather than being put in the "kid concentration camps" of newborn nurseries. Now it is obvious that these nurseries and all their scientific paraphenalia are necessary for the ill babies where mothers took drugs or hyperventilated into long baby-harming labors. But it is equally obvious that these nursery-routines are **not** necessary and can be harmful to both baby and separated mother in the over 90 percent normal and natural unmedicated births achieved through prenatal education and preparation of parents.

Obstetricians make rounds by walking from one patient's room to another and I know of no reason why pediatricians can't check well-babies in their mothers' arms.

The directors of our Academy (AAHCC), themselves the parents of six marvelous children, are reporters of a new concept — the presence of the siblings of the baby and of other interested children at birth. Their teenage daughter, Susan Hathaway, did a study concerning children observing births and gives an excellent presentation of her research at conferences.

As I confine my practice to my cooperating hospital in Denver, I have had no personal experience with children in attendance — we haven't got that far yet in Denver.

Many questions come to my mind and the Hathaways have an answer to each one. It is striking how similar the questions and answers are to my campaign 31 years ago to allow fathers to be present. Should they be prepared in advance so they know what to expect? Answer — certainly. Prenatal education can be **family** oriented, not just for parents. Should children be there if they don't want to be? No, but do they really know what they want? Let them decide after the training classes and films, not before, and an amazing number will change their minds.

Are they sexually motivated due to the genital exposure of the mother? The answer appears to be a resounding **no,** the awe and wonder of the creation of a new individual is all encompassing at birth.

Will these smaller family members develop a deeper bond with the baby as we

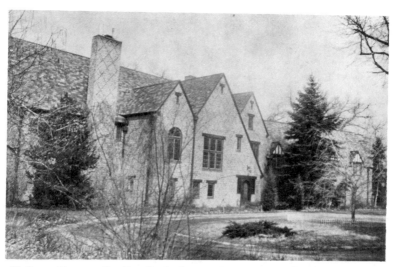

Valleau Manor, the Bradley's home. Dr. Bradley's patients attend childbirth classes here.

have seen happen these many years with the father? Perhaps, time and numbers have not been enough for scientific accuracy, but the current impression is a resounding **yes.** Sibling rivalry is decreased and love for one another increased.

The Hathaway's book is a true first, a true pioneer endeavor to deepen the bonds of the family group into a unit with inter-dependent love.

Like the late Martin Luther King, I, too, have a dream of the future. A dream wherein the 90 percent normality of obstetrics will not be forced to be treated as are the other 10 percent, but all maternity centers will have a home-like natural childbirth unit adjacent to the hospital where sick people are congregated. This unit will be close enough that unforeseeable complications can be handled without harmful delay.

But also that the uncomplicated, through adequate prenatal training of the entire family via trained certified childbirth educators will be giving birth with their families and with midwives in attendance.

These midwives will be trained in normality and also trained to recognize the 10 percent complications so that doctors trained in **ab**normality will be available at all times, when needed.

In my dream all unmedicated mothers will breast feed their babies immediately at birth and keep babies in their arms. They will leave the unit for their homes shortly after the babies are born, as they do now in my private practice.

The 10 percent sick mothers and babies (or complicated ones) will be transferred to the hospital for scientific care of their abnormalities.

This dream is not impossible — it just takes time and determined pioneers, like the Hathaways, to achieve.

ROBERT A. BRADLEY, M.D.
President, American Academy of
Husband-Coached Childbirth
Author, **Husband-Coached Childbirth**
—Harper & Row

A few days before a baby calf had been born and I had seen it. It was I who brought the news of the marvelous event; but then my father and mother forced me to keep out of sight of the field where the mother and calf were, and where I had been but a few moments before. The thing I had seen I dared not talk about or ask about without "deservin' to have my ears boxed."

Even when my little brother was about to be born, we children were hurried off to another farmhouse, and secrecy and shame settled like a clammy rag over everything. At sunset, a woman, speaking with much forced joy and in a tone of mystery, asked us if we wanted a little brother. It seems a stork had brought him.

MISSOURI
CIRCA 1900
From: Lying In By Wertz

WHY WRITE OR READ THIS BOOK

Welcome to our book. This book is not your basic college report with tons of footnotes. It does not deal with lots of boring factual material which has been researched. It does not have a scientific basis which can be examined and argued with pro and con.

This book is being written because of feelings about having children at birth and the authors, all eight of us, Jay and Marjie and the kids — Odell, Susan, Constance, James John, Bobby, and Ann Elizabeth Minniedell (three names for one person) — feel very strongly about this subject. Next question, where did Minniedell come from? It is from her 94-year-old great-grandmother and a beautiful person. I only hope that Ann will be half as beautiful as her great-grandmother is at 94.

We have observed children at birth, done our research, (footnotes are added by Jay — he is the one with the research library on his desk), talked to people, and we have experienced family birthing together. So you see, we are writing and you are reading a book that has some research, lots of personal observation, personal interviews, and lots of personal experiences.

To start with I should tell you that — my husband Jay and myself Marjie — have six wonderful, rambunctious, calm, playful, helpful, happy, healthy children. We have come a long way in our thinking about birth and we have had six very different births, learning with each one. Perhaps if you read this book you will not make some of the mistakes, nor take as long as we did, to learn. Now don't get me wrong. I have nothing against making mistakes and learning by doing. But sometimes it is a painful way. Some people can only learn this way, but at least they learn. Other people may never want to get to the point we are at, and that is all right too. No, I guess I really don't feel it is all right or I would not go to the effort to write this book. I feel very strongly that children should be properly prepared and be encouraged to attend the birth of their brothers and sisters.

I also believe that natural childbirth is the only way to have a baby. Medication should be used only for true medical problems, as a last resort. This is necessary only three to four percent of the time. Breastfeeding is not just a substitute for bottle feeding. It is God's nourishment for a baby. My other prejudices include the family. It is a necessary and holy institution.

Now that you know my prejudices I hope you will bear with me as I am sure you have your own. I feel more honest if I share this with you from the beginning.

Our first experience with birth occurred nine months after we were married;

our first child was born — a beautiful redheaded baby, Odell. Next came Susan a year-and-a-half later, and then Connie another year-and-a-half after that. Although these deliveries were wonderful and my children were beautiful, there was something missing. I was administered drugs that knocked me out. Jay and I kept thinking there has to be something better than this. There had to be another way to have a baby.

As luck would have it, a friend, Karen Osterlund, invited us to attend a lecture in Los Angeles given by Dr. Robert Bradley of Denver, Colorado. He was something else. He said that you do not need medication to have a baby, you can breastfeed your baby on the delivery table, walk out of the delivery room and go home shortly after the birth. And, best of all, the husband should be with his wife at all times.

We were so excited. His words were heaven sent and on my next visit to my doctor I told him all the things that I wanted to do. In Los Angeles in 1965 this was unheard of and my doctor said "no" to everything. I am sure he thought I was crazy. We were crushed. But we still wanted to have our baby together, so we searched all over Los Angeles trying to find a doctor or hospital that would allow us to be together. We had no success. I continued going to my doctor preparing myself as best I could. I took classes, and purchased Dr. Bradley's newly published book "Husband-Coached Childbirth." Jay and I read it together, latching on to every word. It made so much sense.

As the time came close for the birth, I went for my regular check-up and the doctor told me I was four centimeters dilated. (For those of you who do not know, your cervix dilates from zero to approximately 10 centimeters.) The doctor told me I would definitely have my baby this weekend, and this was Friday. Was I excited? Of course.

Monday morning I was still pregnant. Oops! Tuesday morning I woke up, turned to Jay and said, "That's it, let's go!"

We took our kids, drove down to Los Angeles International Airport and boarded a plane for Denver, Colorado where Dr. Bradley practices. It was a foolish thing to do but such a wonderful experience. It changed our whole lives.

I did not require any medication, I breastfed on the delivery table, walked out of the delivery room, and Jay was with me the entire time. The only thing we did not do was to go home two hours after the baby was born like so many of Dr. Bradley's patients. We had never been to Denver before so we went sightseeing instead. Dr. Bradley told us not to come back to Denver everytime we wanted to have a baby, but to return home and get things started. This is what we have done.

We began by teaching classes which quickly grew to six classes a week with 30 couples in each class (far too large a class for personal involvement). At this point we founded the American Academy of Husband-Coached Childbirth, along with Dr. Bradley, and began training instructors in the Bradley Method. Rae Handy was the first Bradley teacher trained and she along with Dr. Bradley and Rhondda Hartman helped us put on our first formal training session.

Although Jay's real job is that of a film producer, we spend much time traveling the country, training teachers, putting on workshops and showing movies for whomever is interested. The birth of James John Hathaway in Denver was such a spiritual experience for me that I really feel it is God's work to tell people that it is possible to have natural childbirth. "Ye of little faith" your body does work! It was not a mistake the way you were built. Having babies may be hard work

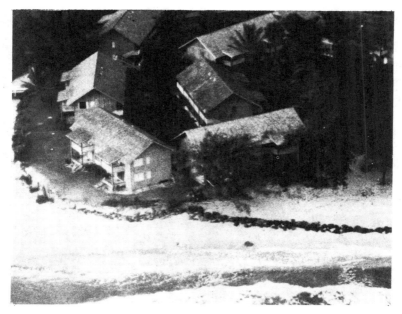

Hanelei, Kauai, Hawaii

and may sometimes be painful, but it can be fun, rewarding, fulfilling and terrific.

The birth of Bobby was another lesson in itself. It occurred on a day when there was a partial eclipse of the sun in Los Angeles. That may not be important to you but I thought it was neat. After we arrived at the hospital the doctor told us the baby was dead, as no heart beat could be heard for 12 hours. Bobby was born fine, pink and crying. I put him to my breast in disbelief and, yet, I knew he would be all right. We called him our "miracle" baby.

The birth of Ann was another matter. We decided to have her at home because we wanted our children to share in the experience. Our good friends, Dr. Victor Berman and his wife Salee, a registered nurse, agreed to attend our birth, even though they normally do not attend home births. We got everything ready, wrote down the rules of the birth that were important to us.

The kids came home from school, we had our dinner and went to bed. About 4 a.m. we woke everyone and said "This is it!" We called the Bermans and some friends. Bob and Jean Kinsella, Steve and Lisa Cushing, Gloria Goold, Debbie Schaffer, Laurie Fowler (Jay's sister), Lucille Hathaway (Jay's mother), Weaver Stevens (our minister) were all there. We showed movies, ran video tapes, played computer games and our labor continued for 35 long hours.

About noon I started to push gently. By four o'clock we asked Vic to check to see why it was taking so long. He checked and said I was almost fully dilated. One or two more contractions and the baby would come right down. Two hours later and no progress made, we decided to go to the Nachis Birth Center. At the center, with two more hours of pushing, Ann finally emerged, her hand and arm presenting before her shoulders. It was a most traumatic birth! I was tired, and so

3

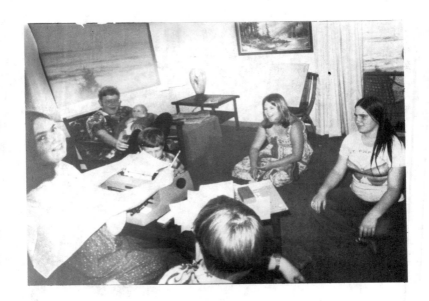

Book writing in Hawaii.

was everyone else. I really feel that I could not have had this natural birth without the support of Jay, our friends and, especially, our children. Prior to this I had considered the effects of birth on other siblings, but this was the first time I considered the effect of siblings on the birth itself.

This experience has led us to write this book to share with you our experiences and hope this helps you.

We feel this book is important. We have trained over 2,500 couples in natural childbirth and have attended hundreds of births, many with children present. We have covered the why's and why not's, how to decide if your child should be at birth, how to prepare yourself and your children, how to handle the actual birth, and what happens after the birth. We will present both the professional viewpoints of doctors, nurses and experts, and those of the children themselves. I hope you enjoy reading this book as much as we enjoy writing it.

The writing of this book occurred primarily on the coast of Kauai in a rented condominium with a rented typewriter shipped from Oahu by IBM. The children are as much a part of writing this book as Jay and I. They have helped by giving us ideas to put into the book. They are our greatest inspiration and deepest critics. They have also helped by writing parts themselves and by keeping quiet, going swimming and babysitting Ann. Ann helped by sleeping, being quiet and smiling. Other parts of this book have been written on the mainland, United Air Lines flights 101 and 114, the volanoes, and beaches of Hawaii, and the beauty of Maui. And, as usual books take longer than you think, so parts have been written in Miami, Chicago, Los Angeles and Tucson, Washington D.C., and more and more.

4

ANTHONY MACK STEWART

You know the Stewarts, David and Lee, as the editors of the NAPSAC books. Did you know that they are also "Bradley" teachers, and Lee is a La Leche League leader. Their first four children — Jonathan, Lora Lee, Keith, and Ben — were born at home. Each of their births has been a DIY (do-it-yourself) and I was honored to be the only 'outsider' ever to be present at any of their births!

The Stewarts lived in North Carolina and it was some project to go there from California with all the cameras, and stuff.

On a cold, February morning, Lee went into labor. It was amazing to watch the

Late First-Stage Labor.

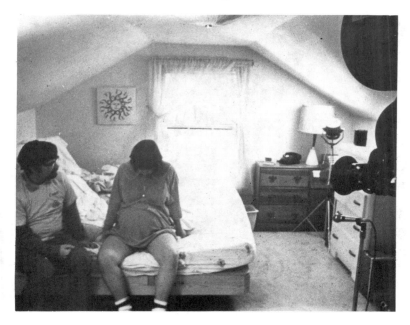

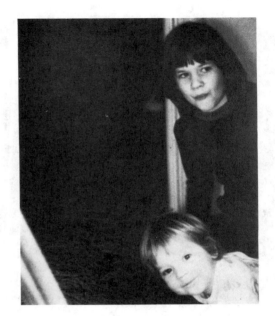

Lora Lee and Ben "checking"

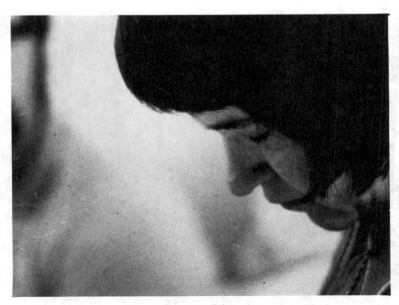

Lee, working.

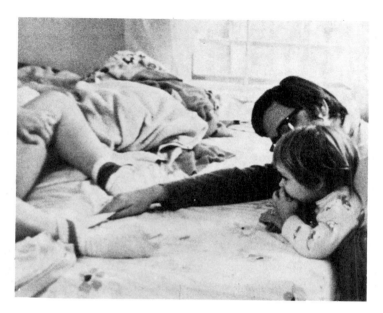

"The baby will come out of there soon."

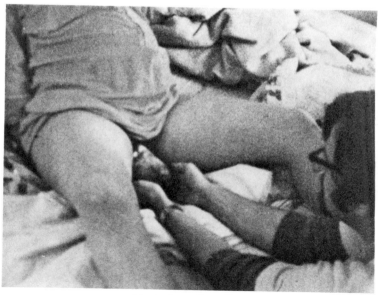

Posterior - Face Up.

7

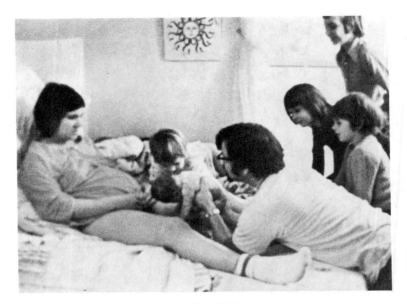

Family Birth.

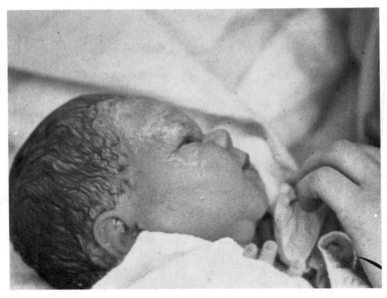

Anthony — with Vernix.

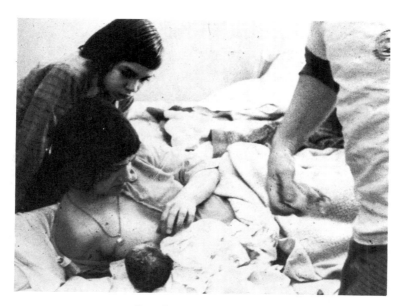

Jonathan says "Hello."

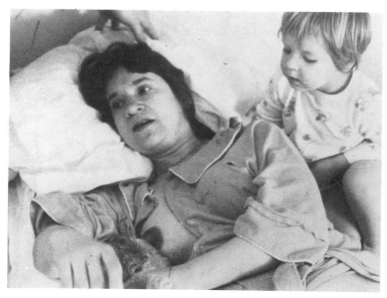

Ben says "Hello."

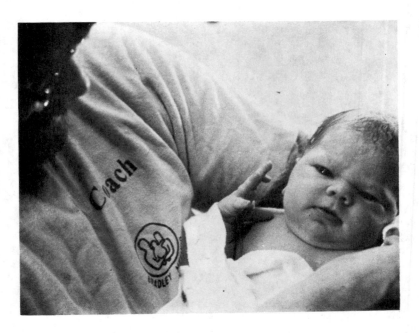

Who says newborns can't see?

other kids care for themselves, and help Mom and Dad prepare for the birth. After a long morning of labor, Lee felt like pushing. Of course, no vaginal exams were done, or needed. As Anthony was being born, our suspicions were confirmed, he was actually born posterior!

I felt it a privilege to be an observer at this event. The results of five unmedicated, NATURAL, uninterfered-with births is truly amazing to see. The Stewart family is just that . . . a family with all the love, warmth, support obvious for those who care to see.

WHY HAVE CHILDREN AT BIRTH?

Children should be present at a birth for many reasons. That is why this book is being written. It is important that they share one of life's most beautiful miracles. It is an opportunity to experience life in reality — the work, the pain, the joy — all at once. It is positive sex education. So often this type of education is negative. Children, at births, learn how to help in positive ways. They also learn how to handle hard work, how to handle pain and discover the rewards that are possible. The birth experience teaches teamwork so children learn how to coach and encourage; how to make others feel better; how to be useful and needed; and how to care.

Bonding at birth is another facet. Is the lack of this bonding possibly a reason for sibling rivalry? Being a part of a whole, learning that everyone must work together to accomplish birth. This experience and learning of the birth process — labor, birth, the cord, the placenta, blood and the new baby — are things children can tell you about, and they do it objectively. They are not afraid of the unknown, as many of us are who have never experienced or been present at an event or happening.

There is no doubt that birth is considered a miracle by most people, except perhaps the so-called modern, materialistic pseudo-scientific society. Our society has taken the miracle out of birth and made it a secret. It is lumped together with "dirty" sex, and very few adults have been present at a birth other than their own. But the miracle still exists. Children are aware of this as much as adults. Children learn to respect birth when they are present and experience it. Birth is no longer a forbidden fruit to snicker and laugh at. It is a responsibility to look forward to when the time is right. Many high school students have commented to me when I show birth films in their health classes that, for the first time, they realize that the miracle of birth holds a responsibility, not to be feared, but planned for and looked forward to. If there is any doubt of this, watch a child during the birth of a brother and sister and see for yourself. It is an opportunity to experience life in reality.

Children learn fast, and being part of a birth teaches them many things they cannot learn anywhere else. Fear and pain go together. Knowledge will break the grip of fear and pain. Children get to see first hand the work and labor of birth. It is real and should not be underestimated.

Having a baby is generally very hard work and this work shows on the mother's face often when she is pushing a baby out. During labor the work can be observed by only people who are sensitive to her if she has been trained to relax. Oftentimes doctors and nurses mistake relaxation, and do not realize how much work a woman is putting out at this time. Children are aware. Children are also keenly aware of any pain or discomfort their mother may be having. This isn't bad if they learn how to help.

Sex and birth are linked together, as they should be. But because they are, sometimes sex is talked about as "dirty" and the reason you avoid it is because the ultimate result is the terrible painful birth experience. When a child is at a birth they see it for what it is. This can be a positive experience in sex education. If we take away all the old wives' tales, dirty stories, misinformation, both sex and birth can become a natural part of life.

Learning to help can be a part of the birth experience for children. They know when their help is really needed. Most children really come through when their help is necessary and this leads to being a part of a whole. Children of all ages can help, some by rubbing their mother's back, kissing her, massaging her feet, taking care of other children. Helping and being needed is a wonderful thing. It gives a person a real sense of belonging and being a part of the family. In interviewing the son of a friend of mine, Roger Kinsella, he said "I felt like I gave birth to the baby. Well, my mother did do some of the work." This feeling carries over into the relationship between children and their parents and siblings.

Handling pain and work are an essential part of life. It does not benefit anyone to avoid them. Children learn to handle their own tasks in life if they can see how adults handle their work. "Hard work never hurt anyone" is a cliche we often hear. Children rarely see anyone doing physical labor. Most adults have jobs that require more brain power than muscle power. Birth, however, requires both. The only work I have ever done that compares with labor at birth is pitching hay or climbing a mountain. Children need to understand this.

Pain is also something we avoid with all of our pills, medications and drugs. If one has a headache today, the way to handle it is to take a few pills and keep going. When having a baby, giving in to medication may be dangerous to the baby. It is necessary to learn how to handle pain in othe ways. Relaxation and tuning into your body is most effective. It is perhaps the most effective tool we have to deal with pain or discomfort. It can be used, not only for childbirth, but for stomach pains, growing pains, menstrual pains, headaches, tension pains, etc. Children need to learn how to handle situations without resorting to pills, medications and drugs when they are not necessary.

Another thing children pick up very fast is how to coach and encourage someone. The act of supporting another human being and inspiring them can be a very important attribute. When you are coaching someone, you must put aside your own doubts and fears and inspire the other person to do their best. Being unselfish in this way can only help build a more understanding human being.

The topic of bonding is a very popular one these days. Bonding between mother and child has occurred since birth began, but is thought of as something new today because of recent research into this area. As a mother, I could have told you that my baby sees at birth. I could have told you that my baby smiles, that my baby sees me and follows and hears. I could have told you this without the thousands of dollars spent for research. Ask my mother. As soon as they mention this to anyone, they are told it is not so, or that the baby has gas, and so on. In the natural course of things, bonding occurs. It is not scientific but just a part of love.

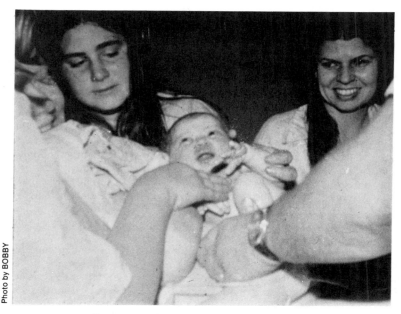

Sue meets Ann. Jean Kinsella looks on.

What about the cases where this does not occur. Perhaps it is because of the interference in the natural process. What do you think a baby imagines when a baby looks into a face covered with a mask? What would you think if it were you? Then most baby's eyes are blurred and burned with silver nitrate. As soon as this is done the baby cannot see clearly.

A friend of ours, a very open-minded person, doubted this. He decided to put silver nitrate into his own eyes. He did this just before attending a birth and had to call in his midwife to catch the baby since he could not see clearly enough. In the State of California the law reads that silver nitrate must be put into the eyes within two hours after birth. I suggest that it might be best to wait the limit of the law and put the silver nitrate into the baby's eyes as late as possible, if the parents decide to have silver nitrate.

Another part of bonding is feeling the baby. In our case this was done immediately. Ann was hot to the touch, slippery, and some might say "yuckie." With tears in her eyes, our daughter Connie rubbed her new sister. Susan also had tears in her eyes as she became acquainted with our new family member. For myself, I pushed so long that my eyes no longer focused. It was with the sense of touch that I realized that we had a girl. All of these factors are part of this peak experience.

Marshall Klaus has reported on much of the work that is being done today about the bonding period between mother and child. I feel this observation could be carried to fathers and baby, and brothers and sisters and baby. It is my feeling that there is a very important bond between anyone present at a birth and the new baby. I have found this to be so when I was at births of people I did not even know.

13

This bond may be carried over to the concept of Godparents. People who will care for the baby if something happens to the parents. For this reason, we chose to have our own children as Godparents, along with Dr. and Mrs. Bradley.

Seeing a new baby being born is a unique experience that few people ever get to witness. Most of the people I have talked with have felt this was a miracle. Perhaps it is the waiting, the watching, the wondering, the disbelief that makes it so wonderful. Susan said to me after Ann's birth, "I cannot really believe that Ann really came out and that she was really alive. . . " Perhaps the first glimpse of a new baby is very discouraging since the first thing you see is the back of the head coming through the vagina. It looks like a mass of gray wrinkles. The first time I saw this I thought the mother's cervix was coming out, or something else. Certainly, not a baby! As the mother pushes, this mass of gray wrinkles comes forward two steps and back one, getting larger and larger. Finally, the head comes out and you gradually see the forehead, eyebrows, eyes that are frequently open and looking around, nose — perhaps a little squished, mouth and chin. The head turns to the side as the baby emerges. Some babies breathe or cry at this time. Others wait.

Next, as the head drops down slightly the shoulders come out generally one at a time. Then the body of the baby slides out. I always thought this felt like delivering a wet, slimy fish — a very nice, wet, slimy fish. If the baby has taken its first breath of air with just the head out, the baby will be pink from the tips of its toes to the tips of its fingernails. If the baby waits to take its first breath after it has emerged, the split seconds that this takes seem forever. Before the breath is taken, you see a wet, slimy, bloody (if there has been a tear or episiotomy) thing. It probably has a white cheesey covering called vernix or baby cold cream. The body itself may be bluish or purplish in color. Tears come to my eyes as this human being begins breathing on its own. I might add that tears generally come to my eyes at births, which makes me a very poor camera person. I leave the camera work to Jay.

The experience of seeing the baby — that new life — emerge, the cord which pulsates and then stops when the Wharton's jelly expands, watching the placenta being born and examining it later — yes, I said examining it later. You would be surprised at how many children want to see where the baby really came from. They love to watch and listen to Dr. Victor Berman's explanation of the bag of waters — the baby's home or swimming pool — where the placenta was attached, and the fetal side, how the blood vessels worked and more. Children seem more interested in this than adults. Perhaps this is because adults have too many preconceived ideas and misconceptions. This can be a real learning experience which may not be available anywhere else.

The most important part of being at a birth is being part of the whole. It takes real teamwork to give birth to a baby. Children can be a part of this. They can help rub the mother's back, break ice chips, answer phones, and so on. Many people today are looking for something worthwhile to do, something that will help others. The experience of helping at a birth does all these things. Learning to be a part, to help, to coach, to give, to experience, to worry, to fear and to love is perhaps a miracle in itself.

JOSHUA SCHAFFER

Kevin was four years old when Joshua was born. He said he wanted to be there, and we wanted him there, too, because we were close as a family. We had also read and talked to other families who had had their children present at their births and were encouraged at their enthusiasm and belief that there was a lot less rivalry between the baby and older ones and a unique closeness.

We involved Kevin with the pregnancy and talked to him about it. We encouraged and answered questions. Since we were "Bradley" childbirth teachers Kevin had had exposure to, and knew how babies were born. He had also picked up our attitude on the "goodness" of birth.

We showed him films and made a point to make comments like "Mommy's baby will come out like that," or "When we have our baby like that, are you going to hold it?" He would ask questions which we would answer. One thing he was a little worried about was the blood. "Why is that baby bloody?" or "Did the Mommy hurt herself?" We would explain and answer. He was encouraged.

Another thing I did was to incorporate ideas from friends who had had children present at their births.

The main idea used with Kevin was to explain how he might get mad about the baby even though he loved it. That there will be times when the baby needs a lot of attention and he might not like it sometimes. In other words, we would allow him to express negative feelings. I think you can push this too much though. I remember trying to say things like,"What if the baby cries all day?" expecting a negative response. He would say "We'll just pick it up and give it "MO," (breast) or "What if the baby messes up all your toys?" "I don't care — I'll just share." One-and-one-half years later he's forgotton ALL about saying that naturally, but at the time he did.

Jon and I wondered if there was a possibility of traumatizing him by allowing him to see the birth. Since there were no "studies," but only our own feelings Kevin's "preparedness" and knowledge (exposure, too) of birth, friends' feedback and experiences convinced us of the goodness and rightness of allowing the family to all be together at the birth of a new family member. I feel also that God has his hand in our children's life and he'll work their experiences for the good.

Another way Kevin was included from the beginning of the pregnancy was to be present when Jon and I went to visit the doctors. The doctors we went to (we switched half way through) were both open to this and would talk to him also.

With Dr. Ford, in the later months, Kevin listened to the heartbeat and the midwife talked with him about various topics.

I feel all of this helped prepare Kevin for the actual labor and birth, so it wasn't foreign or scary for him. Since the attitude given to him was a positive one, he had a positive attitude also.

There were times when he was jealous before and after. But on the whole I, too, can now see an unusual closeness. Nobody messes with his brother. I realize this attitude — the closeness — has to be nurtured after the birth as well. But, again, this experience at the first gives a good starting point. What is the reason for this initial closeness? I think there are a lot of reasons. He was involved with the pregnancy, birth, and so on. He was less apt to feel pushed out of the way. In being there and seeing the birth and holding his brother, I think there is a bonding and imprinting between them as brothers, too. Less jealousy and rivaly is another benefit with the fact that he wasn't replaced, but included in this event. Mom didn't go and leave him and then come back with a "new baby" who all of a sudden is the center of attention!

For the actual birth we made sure that we had someone to watch Kevin and take care of getting him dressed, and so on, so Jon would be free to coach me in labor. My older sister to whom he is very close was there for this purpose and to take pictures.

I went into labor about 3:00 a.m. and Kevin woke up about 8:30 a.m. I was lying on the couch; Jon, my sister and Gloria Goold, a friend who was also taking movies, were there. During the course of the labor Kevin would sometimes sit by me, and rub my leg or back gently. Then he would leave and go outside and play. I remember hearing him through the bedroom window telling our neighbor, "We're going to have our baby today!" At one point he came in and fed me grapes until my cheeks looked like a squirrel's, which got giggles from him. He was so sincere that I kept thinking how much I loved him and was glad he was there. When I got to transition though I remember it irritated me to have him there during the contractions because I wanted absolute quiet and I didn't want to be touched or the bed bumped. I didn't say anything, but Jon picked up my attitude and would suggest that he go play, or go see Jackie (my sister), or play with Jessica — Gloria's little girl. It was nice for him to have a playmate there.

Once Joshua was born and nursing, Kevin came up by our side and Jon, I and Kevin all looked at him. I wasn't aware of his complete reaction until we got the pictures and movies back. I remember he was glad it was a boy. He had insisted it was a boy and that it would be named Joshua. He used to say "It's going to be Joshua and that's AWWWL!!!" Letting him help pick a name was a way of really including him also.

We had Kevin cut the cord and then later had him hold Joshua with skin to skin contact. He said while doing it, "Oh baby, baby, babe." He asked why Joshua was bloody and now a year-and-a-half later when asked about the birth, he said he didn't like the blood, "But that's alright". I've told him a few times why Joshua was bloody and he accepts that.

After a few hours we had a birthday party with cake and a present from Joshua to Kevin. This is sort of a tradition picked up from the Bradley Method and other teachers in the area. It is, I feel, a really nice idea. Kevin really liked that.

As I said, he was jealous at times and now they are starting to have their differences, but there is a special closeness and protection. When Kevin was jealous in the beginning, he never took it out on his brother or tried to hurt him.

16

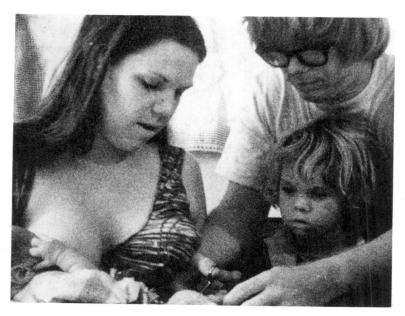

Kevin helps Daddy cut the cord.

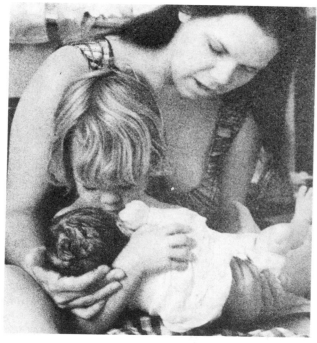

A welcoming kiss for Joshua.

17

He was interested in Joshua's care from the beginning. I still remember looking up one day to see Kevin carrying our two-day-old baby across the room to me — Whew! "Thank you, Kevin," I said as I carefully took Josh from him. There is a closeness!

Here are some excerpts from the journal I kept and hope they may be of interest to you.

July 16 — Jon practices relaxation with me and you like to help. Sometimes you jump all around and make a lot of noise and Jon tells you you're going to have to be quiet when the baby comes. Sometimes you rub my back or feet while Jon talks me into relaxation. Sometimes when I do my pelvic rocks you rub my back too, or bring lotion and rub my feet. Thank you so much, Kevin.

July 25 — Had a baby shower last night — Kevin handed me the presents and said they were all from him. I told him we'd had a shower for him before he was born, too.

July 31 — Kevin has been getting upset and crying more and wanting to play baby at times. I'm trying to give him special time — he's so special.

Aug. 19 — Our son was born today! Kevin cut the cord and held him later and sang "baby baby, babe". He liked eating the cake and getting his birthday presents. He was so glad it was a "Baby Joshua." Later at night I held him and nursed the baby and we talked about "life", a brother — a Joshua baby.

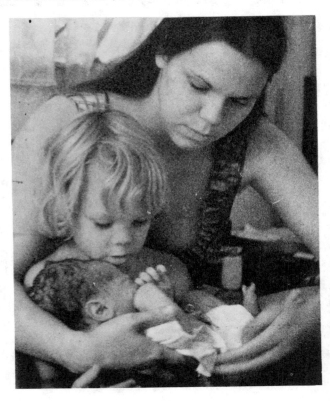

18

WHY NOT HAVE CHILDREN AT BIRTH

There are many objections you may hear for not having children present at birth. As it the custom in our society, these reasons have been accepted as fact. I will go over some of them. I am sure you can think of more.

Negative feelings children might get about sex or birth are one reason I've heard for not allowing children at birth. Modesty of the human body is another. The shock of the process may be too much for some children to handle, or seeing his mother in pain is another fear. Could how or what he tells his friends at school make him an outcast? Could nightmares occur because of the trauma of birth? Might children who are frightened and traumatized never want children of their own? Might they never want a sexual relationship because of this experience? These are very heavy questions. Let's examine them one by one.

Negative feelings about the birth process or sex is a possible reason for not having children at birth. The negative feelings would probably be intensified and reinforced by seeing the birth. It is very much like having someone come up to you and see "Gee, you look terrible. Are you sure you are all right? I saw Joe the other day and he looked like you do now. He died in 24 hours. You had better see a doctor right away." If you felt great before you saw this person, you no longer feel great or, at least, you are not sure you feel great. The negative feelings of the child can influence the birth process itself and the feelings of the child.

Some of these negative feelings may be based on fear of the unknown. This is where classes come in, movies, and so on. Negative feelings about sex may also be based on fear of the unknown. Be careful what you tell your child and how. Some children are looking for simple answers, not complicated ones that overwhelm them.

Another problem lies in the stories they may have heard about birth that are wrong, or perhaps television programs they have seen. One such show was on TV a while ago where children were supposed to see a natural childbirth. The birth scared **me**, let alone my children. My children laughed and turned it off because it was not a real natural birth. The mother was strapped down on a delivery table with two-inch leather straps, her legs were in stirrups, an oxygen mask was on her face, the anesthesiologist was pushing down on her abdomen and the doctor was pulling the baby out. The mother was draped with sheets. The father was there and, the mother had an epidural anesthetic — at least she was awake. There was an IV and fetal monitor hooked up to her. It was more like a machine was extruding another machine part rather than a birth. No wonder so many children have negative feelings about birth if this is what they are told.

Modesty is a family issue. If children are brought up so that they feel it is not nice to see Mommie or Daddy naked, this might be a problem. I don't mean that you have to parade around nude. In our household, if one of our children walk in while we are dressing, it is not a big deal. If one of our children walk in while we are taking a bath, this, too, is just a part of life. In fact we have had some of our most important discussions while I have been taking a bath. I have had a stool installed in the bathroom for the children or Jay to sit on while I soak in the tub. We can talk without interruption of telephones and other things. This is great! I know there are families that feel this is not right, and the birth might be the first time the children have seen their mother undressed. Perhaps this needs real thought if it is a problem.

In our birth I talked to all of the kids about how they would feel about my being exposed in front of them and other people. The only child who had any misgivings about this was Robert. Eight-year-old boys are very protective of their mothers. So we went to the store and bought just the right gown that was full enough to allow birth without exposing my entire body at once, and a zippered front so I could nurse discreetly. When the time came for the birth and I was considerably exposed, this did not bother Robert at all. The time was right and it was all right at this time to be exposed. There is a time and place for everything.

Shock can be traumatic. The birth can be a real shock to someone who knows nothing about it. I have heard stories of children who have hid under tables, behind doors to see the forbidden. These children probably would have been scolded or spanked if they were found spying on thier parents. They undoubtedly did not have any preparation and some have carried guilt feelings with them for life. There is no denying that birth can be a shock to someone who knows nothing about it, especially if they are unwelcome. Might not these same children have enjoyed the experience, if they had been invited, and made a part of birth?

The pain of birth can produce feelings of anger and frustration. It is very hard to see someone you love in pain. Susan, our daughter, told me that she wished she could have taken some of the pain of our birth for me. She felt like hitting someone when I was told repeatedly "just one more contraction" which extended into hours. Some women do not have any pain in birthing and this would not pose a problem. Children do have to be told the difference between pain and work. A woman in labor does a lot of work. Some people mistake this very hard work for pain. The question of pain, discomfort and work can be summed up in one way — it is worth it! The smile on the baby's face, the feel of its cuddle, the smell of its presence is all worth it. Today, three months after the birth of Ann, Susan talks about the day in the future (I hope) when she will have children. Children are such a blessing!

Some children, especially those who tell everyone about the birth, may find themselves outcasts at school with their friends. In interviewing my children, I learned that their friends were not as shocked as their parents. Their friends generally have been interested. Odell says this is because his generation does not have as many "hang ups" as his father's.

Nightmares may be a problem if a child has attended a traumatic birth. This is especially true in situations where communications are stifled. If your child is prone to this, you should discuss it with him and then decide if a problem exists.

Children who attend births may leave with the feeling that they never want children of their own. Children go into and out of this stage even if they have never seen a birth. In interviewing Odell, who is now 16, I asked him if he ever wanted to have children in the future. His reply was "With all the spit-up, changing diapers, carrying, walking and stuff. . . yes."

One student of mine was a person who never wanted children. She felt pregnancy was a time of discomfort and pain and that the birth was even worse. To make a long story short, she met this man, they fell in love and decided the time was right for them to have a baby. Her pregnancy is going very smoothly and she is in class now preparing for the birth in a positive way. If, after watching a birth a person decides not to have a baby, perhaps that is making a decision with more knowledge than they had before.

The fear that children will be turned off to sex is another problem. Odell asked me, when I told him of the topic I was writing about — "What at a birth would turn someone off from sex? What does birth have to do with it? You sure have some dumb topics in your book. I didn't know that being at a birth would cause some problems, but being in this book will cause me problems with my friends." I am sure this can be a problem with some children and should be discussed openly with them before the birth.

All of the problems we have discussed should be looked at and discussed. Some of them may affect your child. Others will be of no consequence to you. It is better to look at them and discuss them before the birth than having to deal with them after. The parents' attitude has a lot to do with the child's attitude. Ask yourself, "Do you really want your children to be there?" Your negative feelings, your feelings of modesty, shock, pain or fear have a great deal to do with how your children will react.

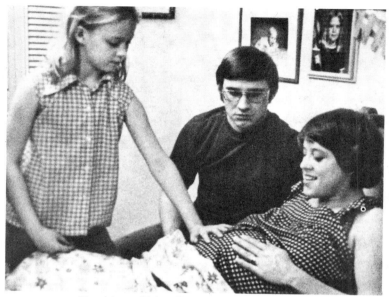

Kerri-Lou, Skip, Jill Skripps — In Labor

JENNIFER SKRIPPS

Kerri-Lou hasn't been at a birth . . . yet

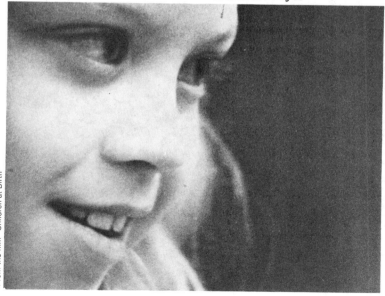

From the film "Children at Birth"

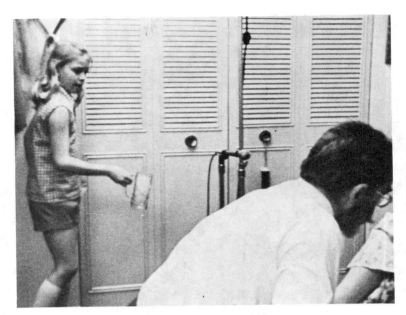

Kerri-Lou Brings Ice Chips

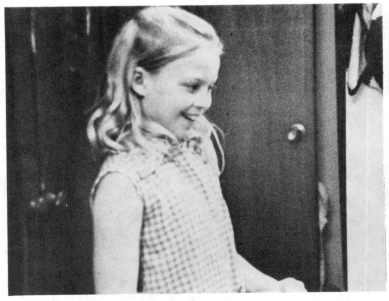

"Can't Wait!"

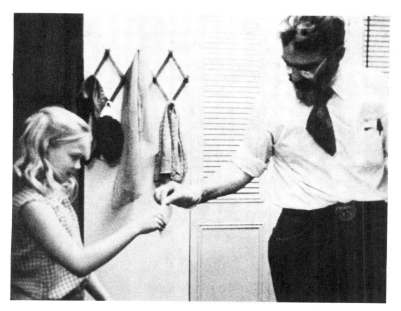

Kerri-Lou Hands (Assists) Dr. Gregory White, (author of Emergency Childbirth).

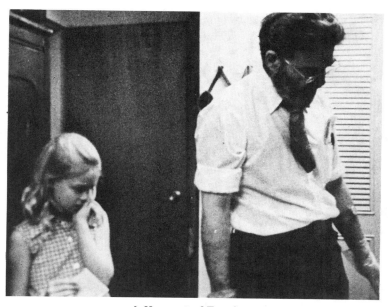

A Moment of Tension

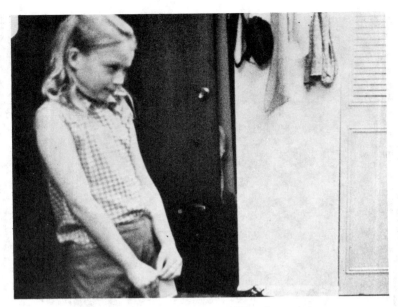

Kerri-Lou helps, by holding her breath . . . too

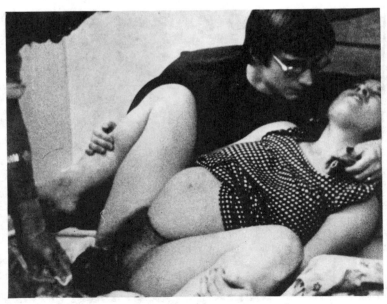

Patience: The Real Skill In Obstetrics

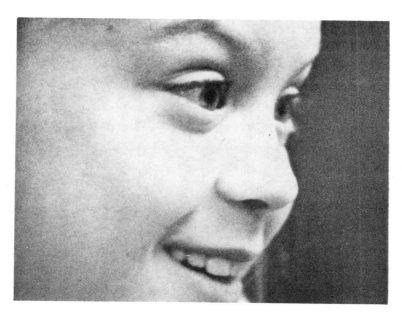

It's A Girl!

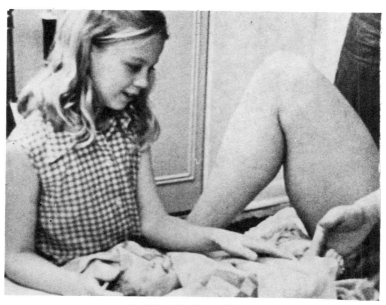

Getting To Know You

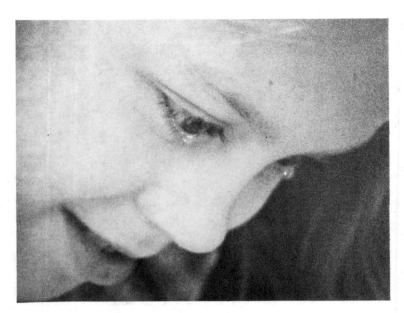

A Tear of Joy

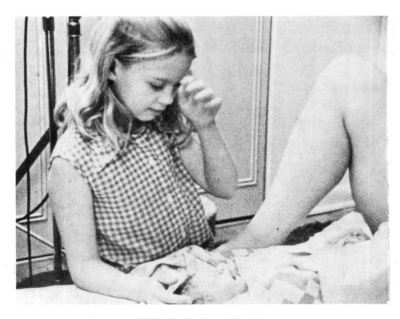

Birth Is So Emotional

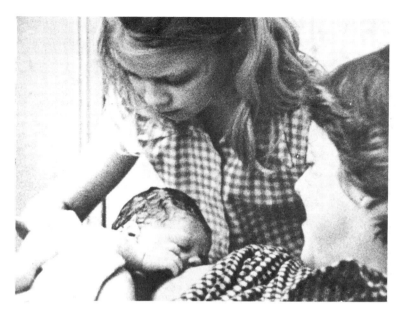

She Feels So Warm!

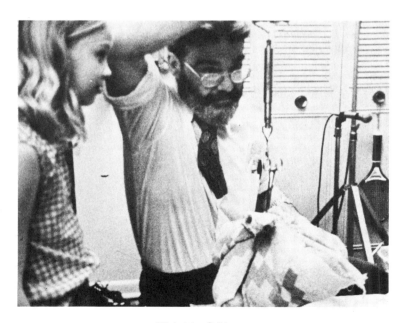

Weight - 8 Lbs.

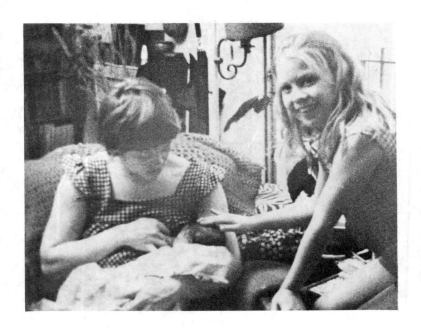

Jill: I didn't think any other childbirth method could be different, but after seeing all the other "Bradley" couples I wondered why I didn't do it that way.

Question: (To Kerri-Lou) What did the kids at school say when you told them?

Kerri-Lou: They thought it was neat, and they wished their mother's would have more babies so they could be there!

HOW TO DECIDE IF YOUR CHILD SHOULD BE AT BIRTH

Having your child at the birth of a brother or sister is something that should be thought through, thoroughly before a decision is made. The decision should be flexible because children change from day to day. Every child is different and they are changeable. They tend to understand what they are ready for, if dealt with openly. The next question you have to ask yourself is: "Are you ready to have your child at birth." And, perhaps, the most important question: "Does your child really care to be at the birth."

Every child is different. Some have great interest in the birthing process. This has something to do with their age. Others may be appalled at the idea of birth. Parents will notice their children's ideas change from day to day. I notice this with mine. You may find your child ready to attend a birth one day and far too silly the next. Different ages have different feelings about nudity. For example, first graders will often break into laughter at the mention of underpanties. Teenage people are also subject to changeable ideas. Parents should be aware of these changes and be flexible in their birth plans. What shocks a child today, may interest him tomorrow.

Children tend to absorb what they are ready to accept. Young children especially are not interested in intimate details of birthing. It's like that old story about the child who asked where he came from. His father, embarrassed but determined to answer all of his child's questions, went into great detail about the birds and the bees. When all of this was over, the child asked, "But where did 'I' come from — Joe came from Chicago." Watch for this trap. When my son JJ was four years old we were expecting the birth of Bobby. I tried hard to prepare all my children for the birth. One of JJ's questions was, "When will the baby come out? How will this happen?" I replied, "When the baby is big enough and strong enough to open the baby door or cervix, it will come out." JJ said thoughtfully, "When I was big enough and strong enough, I was finally able to open the refrigerator door. When the baby is big and strong enough, it will be able to open the baby door."

Openness in the family is another consideration. Does the child know what a person of the opposite sex looks like? To some of you this may seem like a ridiculous question. Some children have never seen their parents or brothers or sisters undressed. Another question you might answer is, "Does your child ever climb into bed with his parents?" This does not mean during sexual encounters. Does the child cuddle in bed with his parents? There needs to be open discussion about the human body between parents and children. When I say discussion, I mean discussion not lecture. Be sure your children understand what you are saying and that they feel free to ask questions in return. The way health classes are today you may find your child knows more about the human body than you do.

Are you ready to have your child at your baby's birth? Please examine your feelings about this. From the mother's point of view: How do you feel about being exposed? Naturally, you do not have to be exposed for your entire labor and birth. How do you feel? Some women want to be nude for the last part of labor and birth. How do you feel about that? Would it bother you to have the birth attendant examine you with your child present? Will you be embarrassed by the gush of water or possible involuntary bowel movement. This does sometimes happen. How will you feel? What about the things that your child might do at the birth.

Let's start with taking pictures. Does this bother you? Or, do you feel comfortable with your child taking pictures. My children took pictures and some very good ones, too. Jay was so busy coaching me that it was very nice to have others to take pictures. Perhaps you should talk ahead of time about what kind of pictures are agreeable to all of you — side views, front views, over the shoulder views. Perhaps you only want pictures after the birth, and so on.

How do you feel about your children talking to others about the birth. Now this can be a real complex question. After Ann's birth my children wore their "COACH" shirts to school and told everyone. I was fearful they would be sent home from school. Most people's reactions were terrific. They wanted to know more. How did it happen that the children were allowed at the birth. There was only one negative reaction. One of Connie's teachers thought that the picture of my nursing Ann was pornographic and she should be sent to the office. As it turned out, many people were interested in the picture and they did not feel it was pornographic. The issue was soon dropped.

Bobby's teacher (at this time he was in the second grade) had asked me to

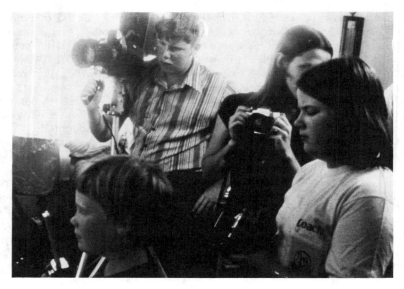

come to school and show Ann to the class. It was mentioned that Bobby was present at the birth and he felt it was "neat." The teacher also felt it was "neat."

Another area that you have to consider is the reaction of the parents of your children's friends to the knowledge of your children. The parents of one of Susan's friends thought it was great Susan knew all about childbirth as she could not bring herself to discuss the facts of life with her own children. In this instance, the family would need to communicate more before the children be invited to a birth.

Another aspect to consider is whether you can face the questions that will

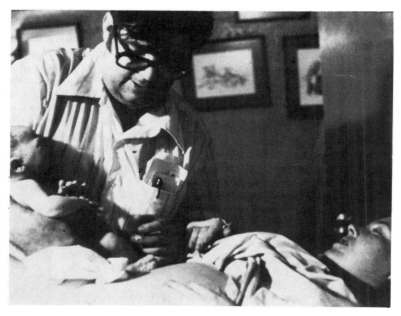

Jay holds Ann minutes after birth (before cord was cut).

arise. One thing that bothers people is being asked questions that are either embarrassing or those that they do not know the answers to. If the questions are embarrassing to you ask yourself "Why?" Then, talk this over with your partner. If you do not know the answers to the questions, find out. This will make for a better relationship between you and your children. It will make for a better birth for yourself. If you know what is happening in your own body, it really helps.

Daddies often have feelings and questions that need recognition. Some men think of their wives as sexual objects. This is fine but how do they feel about his in relation to children viewing the birth? Will the father be embarrassed about other people watching the birth? Will it bother him to be there during a vaginal examination? Will the father feel confident to answer questions children may have? Most fathers feel proud, confident and excited about sharing this beautiful moment.

A mature decision has to be made on all these points. There needs to be a lot

33

of communication. Family discussions are important. Parents should talk between themselves before talking with the children to be sure they agree on this first. If you have any doubts about having your children at the birth, think about it. Discuss it. If you feelings are more positive than negative, then discuss it some more. Your children will pick up on your feelings.

Being an adult is perhaps not the easiest job in the world. After all your talking, preparing and being open, you may find that when the actual birth occurs your child might rather sleep than be there. Or, they might rather play outside or just be there for one quick glimpse and split. Whatever the case, be flexible. Our son Bobby had been at two births at the birth center, both of which ended up being sent to the hospital for complications. He was beginning to feel he was a jinx at births. One evening Salee Berman called me and said, "Bring Bobby down to the birth center right away. There is a birth in progress and the mother says its all right for Bobby to be here." It was a multip, a mother who has had other children, and the birth was sure to go very fast. As births go, this one went very slowly. It was not until six the next morning that the birth actually occurred. Although Bobby had been interested early in the night, he really did not believe it when people had said the baby would come out any minute for the past several hours. Bobby fell asleep. When the time came for the birth, it was a problem waking Bobby. Susan took him outside where it was cooler. People talked to him. Terry was exclaiming between contractions, "The baby's coming! Bobby wake up!" As it turned out, Bobby did wake up to watch the birth for a moment. Then he fell asleep again. However, he was glad he saw the birth and so was I.

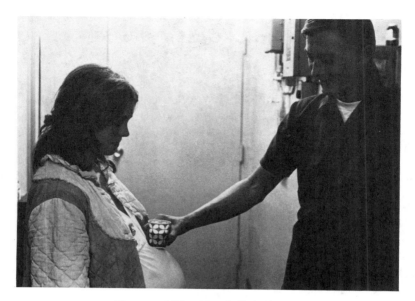

Terry and Wes Hatchell, In Labor

JASON HATCHELL

Bobby Waits Patiently — Drawing "Joy" Flower

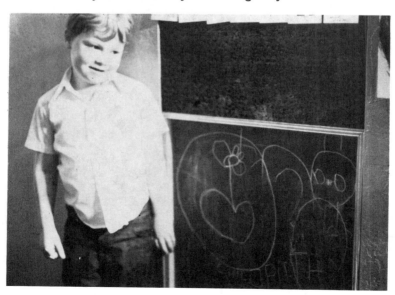

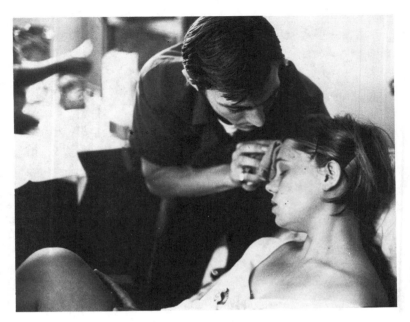

A Cool Wash Cloth

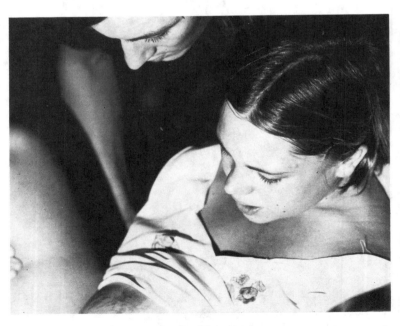

Pushing

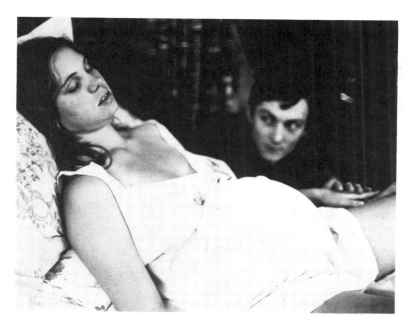

Resting Between Contractions

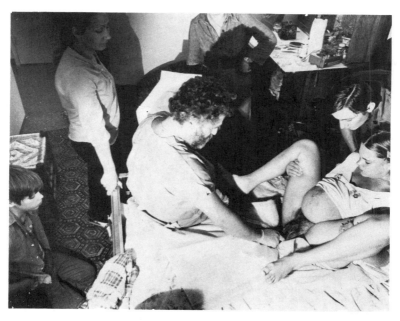

JJ Watches "Crowning"

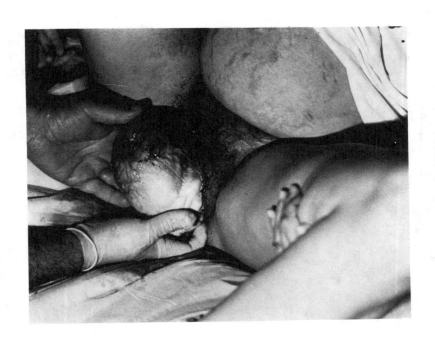

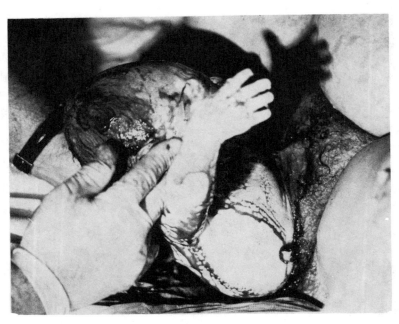

38

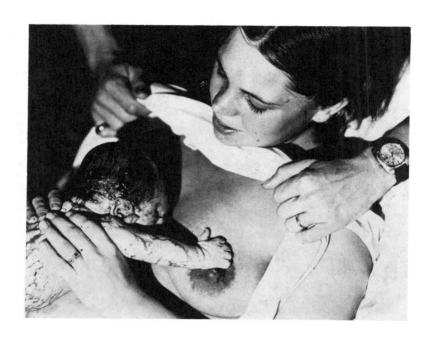

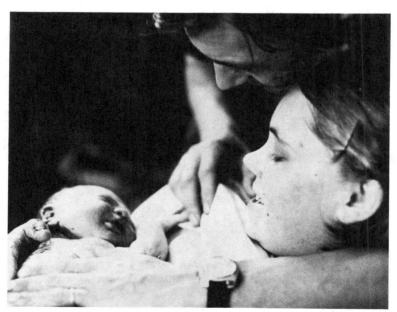

Bobby: (On seeing this picture and being asked if this was the first birth he had seen.) No, this isn't the first . . . I was at MY birth!!!

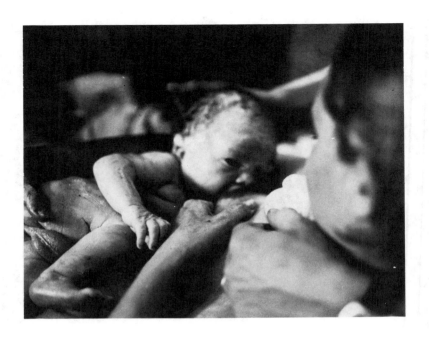

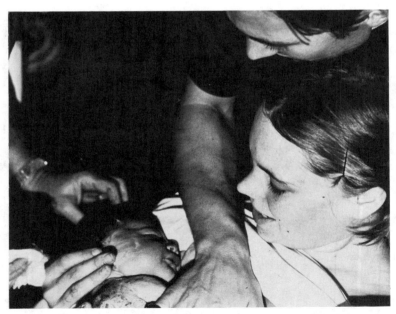

Terry: When I saw your kids at our birth . . . I wished we had brought our own kids, too.

HOW PARENTS SHOULD PREPARE THEMSELVES

Preparing yourself for the birth should start before conception and continue for the type of birth you want during pregnancy. This will include making a lot of choices on where to have the baby, how to have the baby, nutrition, classes, exercises, films, books and what to avoid or use cautiously.

Having a baby is a lifelong commitment to yourself and a new human being. The decision to have a baby should be made wisely and preparation for conception should be made at least three months in advance. Conception should occur when both parents are physically, mentally and emotionally healthy and in top condition. Physical health affects the things one can measure, such as birth defects. Mental health affects the decisions that are made. Emotional health affects the physical and mental well being. The inner peace or emotional climate surrounding pregnancy and birthing is important to the mother, father, children and baby. Infants are born with feelings.

Drugs should be avoided. This includes over-the-counter preparations, food additives, as well as drugs in common usage. If you really have to take a drug, weigh the effects of the drug on you and the baby against the effects of your not taking it. For example, if you have a headache, consider taking a nap instead of an aspirin. The American Academy of Pediatrics, Committee on Drugs has made the statement that, "There is no drug, either by prescription, over-the-counter or food additive, that has ever been proven safe for an unborn baby." Everything you take should be considered. Aspirin affects the blood chemistry. Tylenol affects the liver. Coffee is a drug; it contains caffeine. Cola is a drug containing caffeine. Alcohol is a drug. Smoking is a drug. Tea is a drug. There are many other substances in our daily lives that are drugs and should be considered as such.

At least three months before conception the mother and the father should detoxify their systems from as many drugs as possible. Naturally, in our culture this is almost impossible if you consider what is added to water and what is put into our foods. It is hard to stay away from everything that is bad for you and your baby. But, do the best you can.

The type of birth you want is another choice you have to make. There are basically three types of births — mechanized, prepared, and natural. A mechanized birth is one where you turn your body over to the medical establishment. The type of person who does this is the one who says to her doctor, "Knock me out three weeks before the baby is born and three weeks after." The medical establishment has little choice but to comply with her wishes as this

41

person would probably not ccoperate with any other procedure. These births generally include the use of fetal monitors, IV's, medication during labor, additional medication during birth, forceps, strapping the woman with thick leather straps flat against the delivery table, large episiotomies, long recovery periods, and no breastfeeding with little emphasis on bonding.

A prepared birth starts with classes which are designed to prepare the couple for their birth experience. These classes are not generally geared for unmedicated births although there are exceptions. They tend to apply to the typical mechanized birth but the couples are given information on what is happening to them and the procedures of the hospital during labor, delivery, and after birth. Frequently these couples who have attended these classes are awake, though medicated, for the birth. Most of the procedures used in the mechanized births are practiced here. There is more emphasis on bonding and family awareness with the husband in the delivery room.

Natural childbirth classes, on the other hand, are considered radical in nature. They encourage the couples to ask questions about everything. They do not accept anything as routine. Each procedure should be questioned. Prepping, for instance, has long been accepted as necessary and needed for cleanliness. In looking into this, I have been told shaving the pubic hair started when women came into the hospital with lice. Most women today do not have lice. The hair can simply be washed off for the birth. The hair does not interfere with the birthing process. One objection to not shaving has been that if the doctor makes an episiotomy, some hair might get caught in the repair work. If this happens, the hair can be gently moved to one side and the work continued.

The choices are in the hundreds, if not the thousands. The classes will prepare you mentally with information on anatomy and physiology — what happens during birth and how you can handle it. Other areas covered include: How to deal with all the possible situations that might occur? How to handle a slow labor? How to handle a fast labor? How to handle a not-so-rare, unusual labor. Information is also included on coaching, as well as exercises, nutrition, communication, and so on. For more information on The Bradley Method read "Husband-Coached Childbirth" by Robert A. Bradley, M.D. - Harper & Row.

On the subject of nutrition, good nutrition should start from the time you were born. At least I hope you have had good nutrition since your high school days. This so often is not true. Good nutrition is important throughout your life. What is good nutrition for a pregnant woman?

First of all, you need a balanced diet. Let's start with dairy products. One quart or more of milk every day is generally recommended. Milk can be in the form of whole milk, dried milk, cottage cheese, cheese. What you really need from these products is the calcium for the growth and development of yours and your baby's bones. If you are not accustomed to drinking this amount of milk, start slowly and build up. An extra glass of milk at bedtime or for a snack during the day may be very important.

Two eggs should be eaten each day. Before the flap over cholesterol, this was not considered a problem. Today we get questions about this amount of eggs. First of all, cholesterol may be needed for growth of a new human being. Second, women are not generally susceptible to heart attacks during their child-bearing

THE BRADLEY METHOD YARDSTICK

INSTRUCTORS OF THE BRADLEY METHOD OFFER A HIGH QUALITY COURSE FOR EXPECTANT PARENTS, THESE CLASSES COMPARE VERY FAVORABLY TO OTHER TYPES OF CHILDBIRTH CLASSES' USE THIS BRADLEY METHOD YARDSTICK WHEN CHOOSING CLASSES IN YOUR AREA, HOW DO THEY COMPARE WITH THE BRADLEY METHOD ?

BRADLEY   OTHER

☐ ☐ DO STUDENTS RECEIVE AN OFFICIAL STUDENT WORKBOOK?
☐ ☐ DO STUDENTS RECEIVE CERTIFICATES OF CONGRATULATIONS?
☐ ☐ DO STUDENTS RECEIVE REPRINTS OF ARTICLES.
☐ ☐ DO CLASSES INCLUDE HUSBANDS IN EVERY SESSION?
☐ ☐ ARE CLASSES LIMITED TO 6 COUPLES ?
☐ ☐ DOES COURSE INCLUDE AT LEAST 15 HOURS OF INSTRUCTION?
☐ ☐ ARE WEEKLY REVIEW CLASSES OFFERED FREE, UNTIL BIRTH ?
☐ ☐ HOW DO CLASS FEES COMPARE ? (QUALITY CLASSES GENERALLY COST MORE)
☐ ☐ ARE CLASSES CONDUCTED ON THE FLOOR ? (VERY IMPORTANT)
☐ ☐ DO CLASSES PREPARE COUPLES FOR AN UNMEDICATED NATURAL BIRTH ?
☐ ☐ ARE COUPLES TAUGHT TO "TUNE-IN" TO THEIR OWN BODIES?
☐ ☐ ARE HUSBANDS TRAINED TO BE ACTIVE PARTICIPATING COACHES ?
☐ ☐ IS AVOIDANCE OF DRUGS DURING PREGNANCY, BIRTH AND BREASTFEEDING UNLESS ABSOLUTELY NECESSARY, TAUGHT ?
☐ ☐ DO CLASSES BEGIN IN THE 6TH MONTH AND MEET WEEKLY UNTIL BIRTH ?
☐ ☐ IS CONTINUOUS CONTACT BETWEEN PARENTS AND BABY ADVOCATED ?
☐ ☐ ARE CONSUMERISM AND POSITIVE COMMUNICATIONS TAUGHT?
☐ ☐ IS INSTRUCTOR(S) AFFILIATED WITH A NATIONAL RECOGNIZED ORGANIZATION? ASK TO SEE A CURRENT CERTIFICATE OF AFFILIATION.
☐ ☐ IS INSTRUCTOR INDEPENDENT OF OUTSIDE PRESSURES THAT COULD COMPROMISE YOUR BIRTH EXPERIENCE ?

ARE THE FOLLOWING TOPICS INCLUDED IN CLASSES ?

☐ ☐ EXERCISES
☐ ☐ NUTRITION
☐ ☐ RELAXATION IN EVERY SESSION
☐ ☐ FERTILIZATION AND GESTATION
☐ ☐ TRIMESTERS OF PREGNANCY
☐ ☐ STAGES OF LABOR - OVERVIEW
☐ ☐ FIRST STAGE LABOR - PHYSIOLOGY, PERFORMANCE AND COACHING
☐ ☐ SECOND STAGE LABOR - PHYSIOLOGY, PERFORMANCE AND COACHING
☐ ☐ THIRD STAGE LABOR - PHYSIOLOGY, PERFORMANCE AND COACHING
☐ ☐ RELAXED, NORMAL BREATHING 1ST. STAGE (OTHER TYPES MAY BE DANGEROUS)
☐ ☐ BREASTFEEDING (WHY AND HOW) BEGINNING AT BIRTH
☐ ☐ BONDING - IMMEDIATE SKIN TO SKIN CONTACT BETWEEN MOTHER AND BABY AND NON SEPARATION OF PARENTS AND BABY.
☐ ☐ POST PARTUM CHARACTERISTICS AND ADJUSTMENT
☐ ☐ NEWBORN APPEARANCE, BEHAVIOR AND CARE.
☐ ☐ LABOR REHEARSALS
☐ ☐ ENVIRONMENT - ROUTINES FOR HOSPITAL, BIRTH CENTER OR HOME BIRTHS
☐ ☐ EMERGENCY CHILDBIRTH
☐ ☐ THE FAMILY - ADJUSTING AND WORKING TOGETHER.

THE BIRTH OF YOUR BABY CAN BE THE MOST IMPORTANT EVENT OF YOUR LIVES

CHOOSE YOUR CLASSES WISELY

Your local Bradley Method instructor is a professional teacher or teaching couple trained to help pregnant couples obtain the birth experience they desire. These instructors have gone through intensive training by the American Academy of Husband-Coached Childbirth and are required to re-affiliate each year in order to continue teaching The Bradley Method. This insures you a professional instructor who meets the high continuing education requirements of the Academy. Ask to see your instructors current Certificate.

The American Academy of Husband-Coached Childbirth was founded by Robert Bradley M.D. and Jay and Marjie Hathaway for the purpose of making childbirth education information available. The Academy provides Communications Services, Resource Information, Film Showing, Lectures, Workshops, and National Affiliation for teachers.

For the protection of the public, the terms "the Bradley Method" and "Husband-Coached Childbirth" have been registered. Only those teachers currently affiliated with the Academy may teach the Bradley Method.

AMERICAN ADACEMY OF HUSBAND - COACHED CHILDBIRTH ®   P.O. Box 5224, Sherman Oaks, Calif. 91413   Copyright 1977 AAHCC
B - 250

years. Third, there is much controversy about whether eating cholesterol really adds to your body cholesterol. Perhaps it is your state of tension that really matters.

Next you need several servings of protein each day — fish or seafood, liver, chicken, lean beef, lamb or pork, beans, any kind of cheese, and one or two servings of fresh green leafy vegetables — lettuce or cabbage, spinach, mustard, turnip greens, and so on. Your daily intake should also include two or three slices of whole wheat bread, cornmeal, cornbread or tortillas, a piece of fruit or glass of lemon, lime, orange or grapefruit juice, and one pat of butter.

Other foods that should be included in a balanced diet are a serving of whole grain cereal, such as oatmeal or granola; a yellow or orange colored fruit or vegetable five times a week; liver once a week (if you like it); whole baked potato three times a week; and plenty of fluids — water, juice, and so on. You may substitute proteins if you wish, but be sure your proteins are complete and that you get approximately 100 grams per day. If you substitute, be sure all the elements necessary for a well-balanced diet are available every day.

This is an excellent time to improve the total nutrition of your family — husband as well as your children. Be sure you start the day with breakfast, have snacks available that are nutritious, such as hard-boiled eggs, carrot sticks, celery sticks (try celery sticks with peanut butter). Put a relish bowl in the refrigerator with small pieces of cauliflower, red and green sliced pepper, turnip squares, and so on. Have cubes of cheese, fruits and nuts, on hand as well as hard-boiled eggs. And, of course, that carton of milk ready for drinking. If your children are not used to whole grain breads make half and half sandwiches. One slice of white bread and one slice of wheat. Kids think this is funny but it gets them started eating the whole grain breads. Husbands that are white bread lovers also get a kick out of it.

Here are some sneaky ways to increase protein in your meals. **(see chart)**

If you are really interested in improving your children's diet, check on what kind of meals they are served at school. It may be important to send their meals instead of letting them eat a school-made lunch. A hearty sandwich on whole wheat bread with a piece of fruit, some crunchy vegetables and a carton of milk makes a very good meal. Going out to dinner can be a disaster, or a well-balanced meal. For example, going to McDonald's you could have the plain hamburger, fries and a coke. Your nutritional value would be questionable. If you order the quarter pounder with cheese, and milk, you will have a lot more nutrition.

Another option would be to go to a health-food restaurant. They have lots of goodies — avocado salads with cheese, sprouts, and so on. No matter where you go, think about what you are eating. Would some cheese add something to it? Or, perhaps that extra glass of milk. When at home plan your meals carefully. Have the children help if they are old enough. Have them plan a week's meals and help you with the shopping. You may be surprised at how well they do and you may be surprised at what you eat.

We had some unusual and delicious meals this way. My children kept track of what they ate and also what I ate. If I didn't have my quota of milk by the end of the day, they would bring it to me. They learned how to shop and plan meals. They have always been good cooks. All of this was terrific during pregnancy and especially afterward when I really did not feel like shopping for eight people. My children would go to the store and buy the week's groceries. Everyone in the store

SNEAKY WAYS OF INCREASING PROTEIN IN YOUR DIET

Milk shakes from non-fat dry milk (reconstituted), ice, and flavorings

Roasted soy nuts: buy in health food store or make own. Soak soy beans in water in refrigerator for 2 nights, changing water once (use discarded water for soups or plants). Drain and roast in 300 oven on lightly oiled and salted pan until light brown.

Cheese, cheese, cheese! Add grated cheese to eggs, sandwiches, casseroles, salads, snacks: on whole wheat crackers and celery.

Cottage cheese is the sheapest and best source of protein! Add to gelatin salad, scrambled eggs, casseroles such as lasagna and other Italian dishes, make vegetable and cracker dips out of blended cottage cheese, onions, spices.

Non-fat dry milk: add to hamburgers, meatballs, meatloaf, casseroles, and breads.

Yoghurt: blend with gelatin for interesting fruit salad, use in place of sour cream for dips.

Soy flour: Add to bread (¼c.) when baking

Eggs: keep hard boiled and deviled eggs in refrigerator for snacking, make custard for dessert.

Sunflower seeds: Add to sandwich spreads (chicken salad) and salads.

Wheat germ: add to cereal, breads, cookies, baked goods, serve over ice cream.

Brewers Yeast: increases needed B vitamins too and helps combat fatigue. Good for milk production too.

Liver: best source of just about everything! Cook and grind to combine with hamburger.

Granola: make own from whole grain cereals (oatmeal, 4 grain cereal) wheat germ, coconut, nuts, sesame seeds, sunflower seeds, oil, honey, vanilla, cinnamon.

Combining vegetable proteins to make complete proteins:
Rice + legumes, corn + legumes, wheat + legumes, wheat + sesame + soy beans, rice + sesame, rice + Brewers yeast, beans + corn, vegetables + mushrooms or nuts or sesame seeds.

Beans and Corn: marinated salad of kidney beans, corn, celery, onion and Italian dressing. Serve chili with cornbread. Mexican food !

REMEMBER: Adequate protein (about 100 gr.) helps prevent edema.

DIETARY IRON
Needed for blood manufacture for increased blood volume of mother and for baby. Oxygen carrying component of blood dependent on iron. Also baby stores iron in liver for postpartum life.

Good sources: liver, organ meats, whole grains, beans and peas, corn,

R-495

was so impressed and JJ said he really felt grown up having so much money in his pocket, Daddy waited with the car while they filled two baskets full of the week's meals. A great help!

Here is a chart for you to keep to see if you are getting a well-balanced diet and enough protein. Have everyone in your family keep track of what they eat. I've included a copy of the The Bradley Method Nutrition Brochure to help your family with meal planning.

Sleep and rest are very important to your preparation for the birth. There is nothing worse for the family than a cranky mother. I believe the number one cause of this is lack of sleep. When you are pregnant you need more sleep. If you do not get it, you can become very disagreeable. Sleep during the day if you can. If you have other children this can pose a problem, especially, if they are toddlers who no longer take naps. My solution was to take them into my bedroom and have it child-safe. I would close and lock the door, then place some toys on my bed with the agreement that they did not have to sleep. As long as I was asleep they were not allowed off the bed. They also got great enjoyment from brushing and styling my hair as I slept. This would not work for everyone but it was great for me. Perhaps the answer for you would be to hire a teenage babysitter for an hour or two in the afternoon to take your smaller children to the park. You will be surprised at how refreshed you feel if you get enough sleep.

Exercise is the next topic. For complete information on exercise read "Exercises For True Natural Childbirth" by Rhondda Hartman, AAHCC - Harper & Row. When you attend the Bradley Method classes you will be instructed in the basic exercises for pregnancy. Tailor sitting should come naturally to you. After a while, sitting on the floor will become more comfortable. Children do it all the time. When you start this exercise, as with all exercises, begin slowly and carefully. If you have any questions about any of the exercises, ask your doctor. If you have trouble tailor sitting at first, do it leaning against a wall. After a while you will just sit this way normally. Do your children a favor and encourage them to sit this way. In that way they will not have to learn it when going to classes.

The squatting exercise is next. Again, this is something that children do naturally. When your teacher tells you about this exercise, listen to what she says and do it slowly. Use your hands out in front of you for balance, or try squatting together by holding onto each other's wrists. Don't let go. Another way is to hold onto a door knob and squat. If you choose this method, be sure to walk your hands down the edge of the door gradually until they are on the floor. Keeping your hands on the door knob will not help you learn the exercise unless you gradually bring them down on the floor.

Pelvic rock is one of my favorites. Here again, you should do this one slowly. Get down on all fours, form a box with your hands and knees, and slowly make a swayback by rotating your pelvis. Then tuck your hips under and bring your back level again. It feels terrific. If this exercise bothers you, make sure you are doing it properly and slowly. Most mothers love this exercise because it feels so good.

The sleep position is the way most pregnant women sleep. For those of you who are still looking for a comfortable position, try this one. Lie on your side with the pillow under your head and breast (at an angle). One arm should be behind you and the other arm in front. Both arms should be slightly bent. The top leg should be placed forward. Both should be slightly bent. You can adjust the pressure on the

46

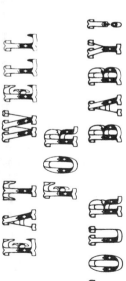

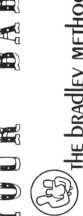

THE Bradley METHOD

wants you and your baby to have the best, safest and most rewarding birth experience possible. For that reason we endorse and teach the following ideals in classes:

1. Natural Childbirth
2. Active Participation of the Husband as Coach
3. Excellent Nutrition, the foundation of a healthy pregnancy
4. Avoidance of drugs during Pregnancy, Birth, and Breastfeeding unless absolutely necessary
5. Training: "early-bird" classes followed by weekly classes starting in the 6th month, continuing until birth
6. Relaxation and NATURAL breathing
7. "Tuning-in" to your own body
8. Immediate and continuous contact with your new baby
9. Breastfeeding, beginning at birth
10. Consumerism and positive communications

You as Parents will have to decide what ideals you have.

Your local Bradley Method instructor is a professional person or couple trained to help pregnant couples obtain the birth experience they desire. These instructors have gone through intensive training by the American Academy of Husband-Coached Childbirth and are required to re-affiliate each year in order to continue teaching The Bradley Method. This insures you a professional instructor who meets the high continuing education requirements of the Academy. Ask to see your instructors current Certificate.

The American Academy of Husband-Coached Childbirth was founded by Robert Bradley M.D. and Jay and Marjie Hathaway for the purpose of making childbirth education information available. The Academy provides Communications Services, Resource Information, Film Showings, Lectures, Workshops, and National Affiliation for teachers.

For the protection of the public, the terms "the Bradley Method" and "Husband-Coached Childbirth" have been registered. Only those teachers currently affiliated with the Academy may teach the Bradley method.

American Academy of Husband-Coached Childbirth - P.O. Box 5224 Sherman Oaks, Ca. 91413 ®

DURING PREGNANCY A WELL BALANCED DIET CONSISTS OF:

Every day of the week you and your baby should have:

1. One quart (4 glasses) or more of milk. Any kind will do: whole milk, low fat, skim, powdered skim, or butter milk.
2. Two eggs.
3. One or two servings of fish or seafood, liver, chicken, lean beef, lamb or pork, beans, any kind of cheese.
4. One or two good servings of fresh green leafy vegetables: mustand, collard, turnip greens, spinach, lettuce or cabbage.
5. Two or three slices of whole wheat bread, cornmeal, cornbread, or tortillas.
6. A piece of citrus fruit or glass of juice of lemon, lime, orange or grapefruit.
7. One pat of butter.
8. Other fruits and vegetables.

Also include in your diet:

1. A serving of whole grain cereal such as oatmeal or granola.
2. A yellow or orange-colored fruit or vegetable five times a week.
3. Liver once a week. (if your like it)
4. Whole baked potato three times a week.
5. Plenty of fluids, water, juice etc.

You may substutite proteins if you wish, being sure your porteins are complete, and that you get around 100 gms per day. If you substitute, also be sure all the elements necessary for a well balanced diet are available every day.

PROTEINS COUNT

MILK 1C	8gm		POTATO	1gm
CHEESE - 1sl.	4gm		RICE 1C (brown)	14gm
COTTAGE 1C	30gm		CORN 1C.	5gm
ICE CREAM 1C.	6gm			
EGG	6gm		PEANUT BUTTER 1C.	12gm
YOGURT 1C.	8gm		PEANUTS 1C.	12gm
			WALNUTS 1C.	13gm
BEEF 3oz.	20gm			
CHICKEN 3oz.	23gm		PINTO BENAS 1C.	15gm.
TURKEY 3oz.	27gm		LIMA BEANS 2C.	8gm.
PORK 3oz.	21gm		NAVY BEANS 1C.	15gm
LIVER 3½ oz.	26gm		KIDNEY BEANS 1C.	15gm
HADDOCK 3oz.	16gm		COLAS	0gm
SALMON 3oz.	17gm		WHITE SUGAR	0gm
HALIBUT 3½oz.	26gm		CARMELS	trace

Resource information for this pamphlet: *Nutrition during Pregnancy and Lactation* from California Department of Health, *Husband-Coached Childbirth* by Robert Bradley M.D. *Nurishing Your Unborn Child* by Phyllis Williams.

SEE THE FILM NUTRITION IN PREGNANCY with Tom Brewer M.D.

MEAL	MONDAY FOOD	Protein Count	TUESDAY FOOD	Protein Count	WEDNESDAY FOOD	Protein Count	THURSDAY FOOD	Protein Count	FRIDAY FOOD	Protein Count	SATURDAY FOOD	Protein Count	SUNDAY FOOD	Protein Count
SNACK														
BREAKFAST														
SNACK														
LUNCH														
SNACK														
DINNER														
SNACK														
SNACK														
PROTEIN TOTAL														

Daily checklist (each day):

MILK ☐ ☐ ☐ ☐
EGGS ☐ ☐ ☐
PROTEIN ☐ ☐
GREENS ☐ ☐
BREADS ☐ ☐ ☐
CITRUS ☐
BUTTER ☐
FRUITS ☐
VEGETABLES ☐
CEREAL ☐

ALSO EACH WEEK INCLUDE :

A YELLOW OR ORANGE-COLORED FRUIT OR VEGETABLE ☐ ☐ ☐ ☐
LIVER ☐
WHOLE BAKED POTATO ☐ ☐

48

baby by bending your legs. Toward the end of your pregnancy you might also like to have a pillow or two under your top leg for comfort.

Perhaps this is the time to mention that you should never lie on your back for any length of time. Not only is it uncomfortable to have the pressure of the baby, uterus and waters on your spine, but it can be dangerous for your baby. I sincerely recommend that you attend the Bradley classes where they will not teach any exercises that makes you lie on your back. If there are no Bradley classes available in your area, then you might attend others, but make sure you eliminate any exercises or positions that have you lying on your back. The pressure of the enlarged abdomen against the largest blood vessels that lie along your spine can stop, or decrease the blood flow through them. This decreases the blood flow to the uterus, cutting down on the oxygen supply to your baby.

As far as the mother is concerned, lying on the back decreases the blood flow to and from the legs to the heart, kidneys and brain. It just is not a wise practice. In

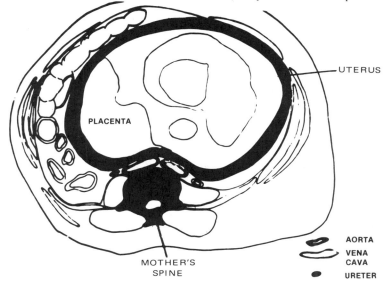

From the film "Obstetrical Intervention" with Roberto Caldeyro-Barcia, MD. Jay Hathaway Productions.

extreme cases, it can cause shock and the mother may pass out just from lying on her back. You should be careful of this during pregnancy. And, it is even more important during labor.

The legs apart exercise is important to tone the abductor muscles in the legs. These are the muscles the enable you to spread the legs apart. It is very difficult to have a baby with your legs together.

The Kegel exercise is next and a very important exercise for life. This exercise is like **not** going to the bathroom. You squeeze the pubococcygeous muscle which goes from the pubic bone in the front to the coccyx in the back. This muscle supports everything above it. As the uterus and baby get heavier, this muscle has

49

more pressure on it. It is important to keep it toned for pregnancy and the birth process. During pregnancy it helps you stay comfortable. Some women have a problem of wetting their pants when they laugh, cough or sneeze. This may be due to a weakened PC muscle.

During the birth, if this muscle is well toned, the baby's head will pass through it when it is high up. This allows the baby to come down the vagina as if it were on a

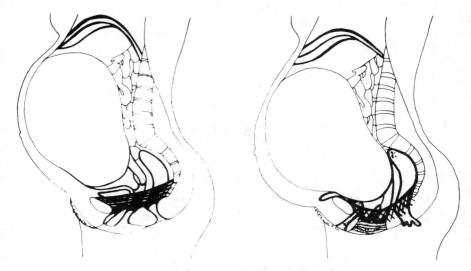

ILLUSTRATIONS BY GLORIA GOOLD, AAHCC

Kegel Muscle in Good Tone　　　　　**Kegel Muscle in Poor Tone**

slide. If the muscle is in poor tone, the baby's head pushes the muscle forward, causing it to tear and bruise. As a result, it could possibly be included in the episiotomy. Another important function of this muscle is that it is responsible for the female sexual climax. If damaged during birth this could cause sexual problems after birth. As you can see, it is important to keep this muscle toned.

Do your Kegel exercises regularly. You should work up to about 200 a day. That may sound like a lot but if you would do 10 Kegels every time you go to the bathroom you would be up to 200 by lunch. Ask your Bradley teacher for Kegel stickers to help remind you to do the exercises.

Perhaps now is a good time in this book to talk about sex. The medical establishment has differing views about sexual encounters during pregnancy. Most of the doctors I know feel that sexual relations are beneficial during pregnancy up to the time the bag of waters breaks. This should be in the second stage. It is important to realize that not all pregnant women have the same sexual desires during pregnancy as when not pregnant. Some women find that their sexual desire increases during pregnancy, others find their desire decreases, and there are some that fluctuate. At one time there was a theory around that if you were carrying a girl your sexual drive would lessen and, if a boy, it would increase

50

because of the hormones. One day a friend of mine called and said, "Marjie, I am going to have twin boys." As you may have guessed, she had a girl. So much for theories!

You should remember that the vaginal area is engorged with extra blood and is extra sensitive. Care should be taken to be gentle. This might be a good time to try different positions so that the mother would not have to be on her back. The side position of the hands and knees position might be more comfortable for you. Above all, it is important that the pregnant couple talk about their desires. Some men feel that it is their job just to take a cold shower and be quiet. This should not be the case. Talk about each other's desires and try to meet them.

The next and probably the most important exercise in The Bradley Method is relaxation. Learning how to relax is the key to the Bradley Method and to a comfortable birthing experience. If you are tense you get into a cycle of tension causing fear which leads to chest breathing, which leads to panic, which leads to tension, and the circle goes round and round.

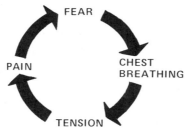

There are three types of relaxation which I want to discuss. Number one is mental relaxation. This relaxation has to do with what you are thinking, how you feel, and what your environment says to you. Jean Kinsella, AAHCC, a Bradley teacher and her husband, are educational consultants to the Academy, have done an exercise on mental relaxation somewhat like this. (Imagine that she is saying this to you.):

"Picture something pleasant that you once experienced. (Early childhood, courtship, something the two of you did together, a vacation, a holiday, and so on.) Now we are going to go back to that particular time and experience it once again. Try to remember what it looked like; who was there; what they were wearing; what colors you remember; foreground, background; shapes; sizes and so on. (Between each category, give a time of silence to permit maximum experience.) Now, what **sounds** did you hear? Voices? Music? People moving about? Outdoor noises like wind, water, rain, etc.? What **smells** do you associate with this scene? Food? Perfume? Ocean air? Pine trees, etc? Do you associate any **tastes** with this experience? Were you eating? Now let's explore the sense of **touch.** Was it cool or warm? Were you standing or sitting? Did you touch any person? Any objects? Try to re-experience the smoothness, roughness and so on?) Now try to recall your **emotional** climate at the time. Happy? Serene? Excited? Anticipating? and so on." (Give additional time for total recall.)

This type of exercise can be done by one member of the family doing the talking and the rest concentrating on the subjects. Another way to do this is to take a family experience and have everyone think about the same thing. The atmosphere should be calm, relaxed and pleasant. The room should be comfortable with the lights dimmed. If you have very young children, this may not be the thing to do as they may not have the attention span for it.

Another exercise the whole family can do is be aware of muscle tension. This exercise relates to physical relaxation. Sue and Gary McCutcheon, AAHCC, authors of "The Birth Team," Academy Publications, demonstrated this one to me. Lie on your side on the floor in a relaxed position. Now observe and release as someone talks you through this.

Tense your face a lot. Tense your shoulders a lot. Tense your tummy a lot. Now release. This time tense your face a little. Tense your shoulders a little. Tense your tummy a little. Now release. Think about these areas and release a little more. Release a little more. Release a little more. Relax. See how you can release a little more each time even though you thought you had released in the beginning.

Tension and relaxation of different parts of the body is another effective technique. Get on the floor with pillows supporting your body comfortably. Make sure you are in the correct side relaxation position. If your arm bothers you in back, bring it to the front. The most important thing is that you are relaxed. Now "coaches" listen carefully. The person on the floor should follow my instructions. This can be done with a group pairing off. One person should be the coach; the other pretend they are the pregnant person. One person should talk the other through. Now get as relaxed as you possibly can. Tense your right foot by bringing your toes up toward your head. Do not point your toes during pregnancy. (I do not know why but pointing your toes often causes leg cramps.) Place your hand on the foot and feel the tension in the foot. Relax this foot while the coach feels the relaxation come over the foot. Massage the foot so that it is even more relaxed.

Now tense your left foot. Coaches feel this tension. Relax the foot. The coach feels the foot become relaxed and massages the foot so that it becomes more relaxed. Now do this same procedure by tensing the right leg. Relax. Tense the left leg. Relax. Tense the right hand and arm. Relax. Tense the shoulders — feel all the tension in your neck and shoulders. Relax. Tighten up your facial muscles. Relax. Now concentrate on your muscles being loose, limp and relaxed. Relax for a few minutes and feel yourself sink into the floor. As you practice this you will be able to become more and more relaxed.

Another relaxation exercise can be done with everyone on the floor except the person reading. Lay on your side and relax. This time tense and relax different parts of your body as we did before. However, there will be no massage because everyone is doing it. Tense your right foot. Relax. Tense your left foot. Relax. Tense your right leg. Relax. Tense your left leg. Relax. Tense your right hand and arm. Relax. Tense your left hand and arm. Relax. Tense your shoulders — feel the tension in your back and neck. Relax. Tighten your facial muscles. Relax. Now let yourself sink into the pillow. Let yourself become more and more relaxed. Sink into the floor. Feel your body become heavy and relaxed. Think about the baby in the uterus. (If you are not pregnant, you will have to imagine this.) The baby is warm, comfortable, safe and relaxed. Think about this comfortable feeling. Now let this feeling flow through your lower back and spread down your hips, relaxing your legs, your knees, calves, ankles, feet and toes. Imagine this warm, comfortable feeling and let your body just become loose, limp and relaxed.

Now starting with the uterus again, feel the baby and how warm, comfortable and relaxed it must be floating in the amniotic fluid, safe and protected from the environment. Now let this warm, comfortable feeling go through your lower back. Feel it spread up your back relaxing every vertebra in your spine as it slowly sends warmth from vertebra to vertebra, finally reaching the back of the neck and shoulders. Concentrate on this spot for a moment. Let the warmth penetrate this area, especially releasing the tension that can build up during the day. Then the muscles go loose and limp. Feel your neck become warm, comfortable and relaxed. Now let this feeling come up the back of your neck, over the back of the head, down the forehead, relaxing the eyebrows, eyes, nose and mouth. The eyes should be closed and the mouth slightly open. Lie there for a few moments and allow your whole body to become loose, limp and relaxed. Think about your hands becoming loose, limp and relaxed. Let your mind absorb this feeling so that you can recall it whenever you want to.

Rubbing the back can be another way of relaxing each other. Pregnant women have special needs when it comes to rubbing the back. First of all, the back has extra strain on it when you are pregnant. The lower back especially has extra pressure. Ask your wife how she likes to have her back rubbed and where. During labor you may find that the coach may rub the back for hours, or you may find a woman in labor who may not want to be touched at all. You never know how pregnant women will react so be ready for anything.

Some women like the palm of the hand placed firmly on the lower back and pressure applied to this area. The pregnant woman will show you where this feels the best. Some women like to have the hand moving in a circular motion as the pressure is applied. Others like to have you make fists out of your hands and apply pressure on either side of the spine. Sometimes they like the palm of the hand placed at the base of the spine and pressure applied in an upward motion. The pressure should be to the degree that it is comfortable for the mother. Everyone in the family can help in this back-rubbing exercise. If the mother is in labor for 12 to 15 hours, which is average, everyone can have a turn rubbing her back. You also might want to apply some lotion to make the rubbing of the back easier.

Ask your children how they like their backs rubbed. Touching can be relaxing and loving. The techniques for relaxation should be used by all family members. It has little value to teach the mother how to relax if the family members are saying in a tense, tight voice "REE-LAX." This only leads to tension for all concerned. When you practice these and other relaxation techniques that you will learn in the Bradley classes, change roles. Let the child and the father play the part of the pregnant mother. This will help each person appreciate the role of the other.

Because of the emphasis that has been put on breathing in childbirth, I feel that it needs an explanation here. **The Bradley Method does no emphasize breathing.** We do insist that you continue to breathe during your entire labor. Our emphasis is on relaxation. The normal breathing for the human being is abdominal breathing. This is what should be done in labor. Other perspiring mammals use abdominal breathing for their labor and that is what the Bradley Method is based on — the observation of the other perspiring mammals. Other types of breathing have undesirable consequences and aren't **natural.**

Classes are an important part of your preparation. It is important how your choose your classes. First of all, I feel the Bradley classes to be the very best, (but, then I am a prejudiced person.) Make sure your instructor is officially affiliated with

The American Academy of Husband-Coached Childbirth. These teachers have had intensive training and most have had babies this way themselves. Official Bradley teachers are independent teachers and do not compromise their classes for anyone. Beware! As the Bradley Method becomes more popular, there are more and more imitations. Some people say they teach part Bradley, or Bradley-Lamaze classes which, it has been said, is like having a baby with one eye open and one eye closed. There are many important differences and the things that Bradley Method does not do are as important as those they do, such as breathing, keeping the eyes open during a contraction, and tuning into your body instead of turning away. Adding to the Bradley method does not make it better, it diminishes it. The Bradley Method is simple, honest and natural. If you attend a class that is any different, it's not Bradley.

Films! Films! Films! There are so many films to be seen today. See as many as you can and take your children along. If you are going to have your children at the birth I highly recommend you see "Alternative Childbirth," or "Children at Birth," which show several births with children present and interviews with some of them.

Other films that might be of interest are: "Childbirth for the JOY of it, Part I and II," "Happy Birth-Day," "Nutrition in Pregnancy," "Breastfeeding for the JOY of It," "Bradley on Birthing" and "Cesarean Childbirth." All of these films were produced by Jay Hathaway Productions and, of course, I feel they are excellent. We wouldn't make a film if we did not think it was great.

Other films you might enjoy are: "First Days of Life" available from many Right-to-Life Leagues and "Amazing Newborn" available from Case Western Reserve University. There are many other films on "Natural Childbirth" that are really **medicated** births, but because the baby was born vaginally instead of by Cesarean it is called "natural". Be sure! If the film does not say "medication was not used for labor, birth or delivery," do not assume this is so.

Another decision for parents to make who want their children at the birth is where to have the baby. The choices seem to be the hospital, the home — attended and unattended, or the birth center. A few hospitals are now allowing children at births. One hospital I know that allows children at births is in Fort Bragg, California. Dr. Michael Goodman allows children at births and has been written up in "OB/GYN News." These births seem to be relaxed and comfortable. The incidence of infection was no higher and births seem to be quite successful. I hope that other hospitals will start permitting this also. There is nothing in the California State Health Code, that prohibits children from attending births. Individual Hospitals seem to make these policies and **can** change them. The hospital vs. home-birth question is a very hot issue. Both sides have their points. The home is definitely the most comfortable and, if proper precautions are made, may be very safe. This means first of all not interfering with the natural process of things. Most complications of birth occur when nature is disturbed, such as inductions, breaking the bag of waters, vaginal exams, and so on. These things should not be attempted at home. (My feeling is that they should not be attempted anywhere else either unless there is a true complication which necessitates it.) Hospitals are generally believed to be the safest place to have a baby but it has never been proven. Few people think about the dangers of hospital births. It is true they have the most equipment, the most available and trained personnel, the most machines, the most techniques available. But these facilities are a potential

54

danger to a natural birth in themselves. The most dangerous thing you can do in a natural birth is to interrupt the natural process. Being in a hospital it is tempting to use the machines, the equipment, the personnel and techniques available. The fact that there are so many people there, also represents a danger. People mean germs; germs that have grown immune to normal bacteria and extermination means. These bugs, so to speak, have become immune and represent a danger to you and your baby. The most notorious of these is the staph infection. This can occur to the mother and to the baby. Almost every major Hospital, Nursery, or OB Unit has been closed down at one time or another when the patients contracted staph infections. These infections can kill. Beware of the hospital births. They not only have safety factors, but dangers, too. On the other hand, home births also have their good and bad points.

Remember, when YOU choose between the home, hospital, or the birth center, you are not choosing between safety and risk. You are choosing between risks; each minimal, but each very real. None of these alternatives have been PROVEN safest. In fact, none are entirely safe; each has its own special risks and benefits. You must weigh them carefully and choose between them!

The third choice is an unmedicated childbirth center (UCC). These are hard to find since so many places are now calling themselves "birth centers." There are a number of questions you should ask about a "birth center." Is it in or out of the hospital? If it is not in a hospital, what facilities does it have on hand? What arrangements do they have to transfer you to a hospital, if necessary? How do you get there? Ambulance or drive yourself? Who will attend you in the hospital? Will your children be allowed at the "birth center?" Will they be allowed at the hospital? Has the "birth center" ever had an infection? Do they do Gyn examinations in the same room as the birth may occur? What kind of staff do they have? Will the doctor be present, or only on call? How will financial arrangements be made if you have to transfer to the hospital?

Birth centers in the hospital are perhaps the most popular now and may or may not be unmedicated childbirth centers. If you hospital has an UCC, here are some questions you should ask:

Is there an anesthesiologist on duty?
Does he charge if he is not used?
Is blood available if necessary?
Is there a lounge for the children to play in?
What is their Cesarean rate?
What is their infection rate?
Does the baby have to go to a nursery?
When is silver nitrate used? Can you refuse it?
Where are emergency C-sections done?
What experience has the staff had with unmedicated births?
What experience has the staff had with children at births?
Are you a pioneer?

I feel it is important that the whole family have a chance to tour the UCC before the birth so that everyone is at ease.

Birth Attendant: Choosing your birth attendant is very important to everyone at the birth. The physical needs of mother and baby are perhaps the first consideration. Are you going to choose a doctor? If so, one choice is an obstetrician who can do everything from unmedicated births, forceps, and C-sections. Ask to see your doctor's credentials. Is your doctor a Board Certified Obstetrician? This type of doctor can do most anything concerning the birth and generally turns you over to a pediatrician for the care of the baby. Family-practice physician is another choice you have. This doctor generally stays away from complications, referring them to an OB. He can take care of the whole family, including the new baby after birth. Your children may feel more at ease if this person has been their doctor over the years. Another alternative that is now available is midwives. These come in two types — nurse-midwives and lay-midwives. Nurse-midwives generally have more medical training, charge more money and may have better back up with a hospital or doctor for complications. They deliver mostly in "birth centers," generally in hospitals. Lay-midwives generally have more practical experience catching babies, but may lack medical training. No matter who you choose to be your birth attendant, make sure the feelings between you are nice. Check out their credentials. Don't just take their word for them. Ask how many births have they caught? What percentage were unmedicated? What percentage of episiotomies have they done? Do they know how to catch a baby without doing an episiotomy? How do they feel about having children at the birth? Will they take time to answer questions? The person who attends your birth is there to help you, but the responsibility for the birth is always your own. Even if you have a million doctors, nurses or midwives present, you are the one who will have to raise and live with your child. Let your birth attendant help, listen to his advice, but make the decisions yourselves. You the parents have the ultimate responsibility.

Be Prepared: This is the Boy Scouts' motto but should also be the motto of everyone expecting a baby. I am now going to list some things I feel you should think about and resolve before your baby is born. Some of these items are only for emergency situations but you should be prepared for emergencies. Answers to these questions will be different in different communities.

What doctors will assist in births should you have your baby at home or not make it to the hospital?

What prenatal care are you getting? Is it adequate? Do you understand why things are done?

Where can you receive emregency care?

Do you have paramedics? Do you have ambulance service?

What is the difference?

Does you hospital have an emergency room?

Who is on staff? What is their knowledge of obstetrics?

Is the emergency room open 24 hours a day? Is a medical doctor on duty at all times?

Does a hospital closer to you have a 24-hour-a-day emergency service? Will they take you if your doctor does not have privileges there?

What is the charge?

Where can you get a prescription filled in the middle of the night?

Where can you get lab work done during the day? Night?

Where can you get X-rays?

What is the difference in cost between having these services done during regular hours and at night?

Who do you call in an emergency? Who do you call if the mother or baby dies? Where can you get a birth certificate?

Do you have day and night phone numbers for your birth attendant? Emergency hospital? Police? Ambulance? Paramedics? Pharmacy? Pediatrician? And any others you can think of.

Do you have helicopter service available in an emergency?

Where is the closest Neonatal Intensive Care Unit? Do they have rooming in?

Where does a paramedic take you in an emergency? Will they take you to a private hospital?

Where can you receive legal aid?

What are your hospital's policies? How can changes be made?

Will your pharmacy give you the package insert?

These are some of the things you should consider, and get answers to.

Communications: This is so very important in preparing for a birth. In the Bradley Method we try to have each couple work on communicating with each other and with their medical team. If your children are going to be at your birth, communications should include them also.

First of all husband and wife need to communicate with each other about the birth, their expectations and fears. Next I feel you need to communicate with your children about the same things, and early in pregnancy find a doctor with whom you can communicate with openly. Here are some communications techniques you may use with your children.

Ask your children to talk about how they feel the birth will progress. If they are old enough, it is fun to have them write out and put in the baby book.

Put open ended sentences on 3x5 cards. Spread the cards on the floor, taking turns having each person take a card and read it and say whatever comes into their mind. Small children may have to have someone else read the card or, if they are too young, this game might not be appropriate. Some questions you might put down could be: What I want others to do for me during the birth is. . . What I expect to enjoy the most about labor and birth is. . . What scares me the most about having this baby is . . . I think labor will be mostly. . . When I think about the birth I usually. . . The idea of touching a new baby makes me feel. . . The thing that bothers me that I have not discussed is. . . The biggest change this baby will make in my life is. . . Watching movies about birth makes me feel. . . The thing that scares me most about the baby is. . . The thing that I feel I will enjoy most about the baby is. . . The sight of blood makes me feel. . . The thing I dislike most about babies is. . . When I think about pain in labor I . . . When I think about handling pain with relaxation I . . .

Each person may have entirely different answers to these questions, and each answer should be accepted as there are no right or wrong answers to these questions. Give each person a chance to add to the original answer by asking if anyone has any other answers to the same question. Add your own questions.

Pass our 3x5 cards and have each person write down 10 things that relax them. Discuss.

Pass out 3x5 cards and have each person answer the following questions. Where do you tense up first? Where do the other members of the family tense up first? Where do you like to be touched? Where do you not like to be touched? Discuss.

Use one discussion time to discuss fears and what if's. How would you feel if: The baby is not the sex you think it is? What if the baby is deformed? What if the baby dies? What if labor takes a very long time? What if after all this planning the baby comes before anyone gets home? And more.

Pass out cards and ask questions and discuss the following:

1. How do you like your back rubbed, scratched, pressured, tickled, and so on?

2. What do you like to touch, feel, smell, and see?

3. List five things you want to do in labor.

4. List five things you want to do for someone in labor.

See movies together on birth. Read books. Talk to other families who have birth together.

Labor rehearsals are very important so that everyone knows what to do if they are called on to coach. Practice the labor rehearsals you learn in class at home, letting the children who are old enough to play the role of coach. Also talk about what each person's role is. Perhaps one older child will be responsible for a younger sibling. Perhaps someone is in charge of pictures, someone else phone calls, and so on.

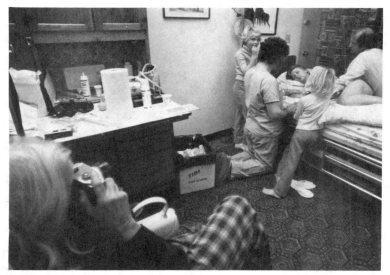

Grandma takes pictures as Steve & Jeri labor. Dr. Berman, Kari (9) and Kris (5) help, too!

SIRI HARRISON

Relax, Mommy.

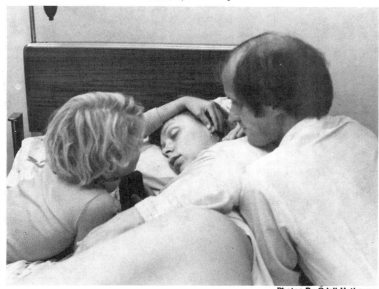

From the film "Children at Birth"

Photos By Odell Hathaway

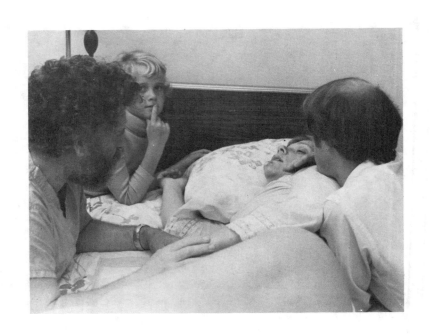

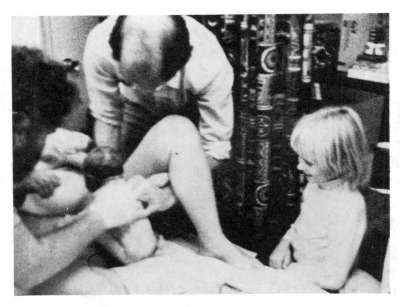

Loving Hands

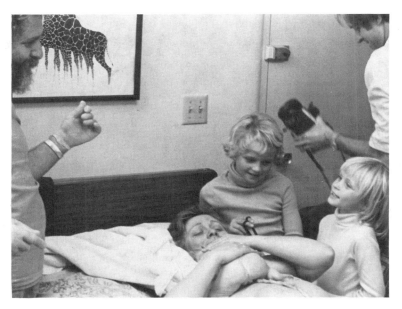

"Aren't you ever going to wash it?"

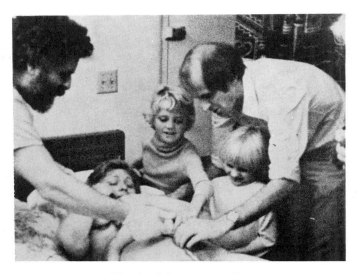

The cord does pulsate!

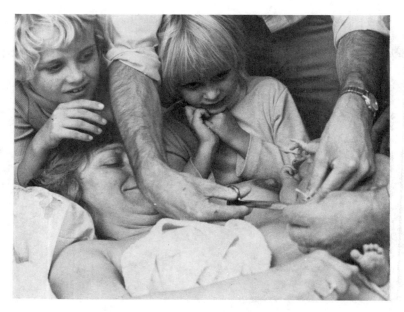

"All Free"

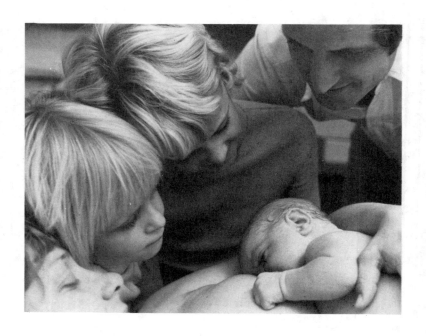

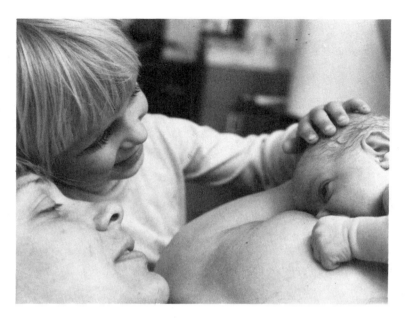

Making a Bond of Love by Touch.

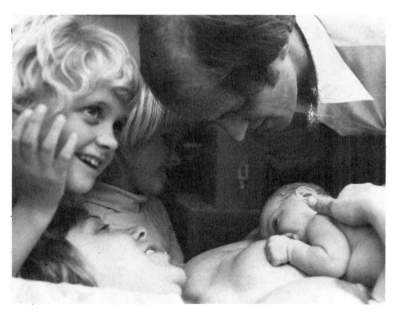

A Family From the Beginning.

CONSUMERISM
(Choices)

"Rarely are mothers taught, in hospital-based classes, how to cope with the hospital and its personnel in a manner which maintains the parents' control of their childbearing experience.

The recognized success of parents prepared by the Bradley Method is, in my opinion, largely due to the Bradley instructor's emphasis on teaching parents how to cope tactfully, but forcefully with the hospital environment."

> Doris Haire, speaking at
> International Society for
> Psychosomatic
> Obstetrics and Gynecology
> Chicago, Illinois, April 1976

"It's not nice to fool Mother Nature."
> Robert A. Bradley, M.D.

When Marjie asked me to write this chapter . . . on consumerism ... I hesitated for a moment. I wondered what a chapter like this would be doing in a book about "Children At Birth." But, thinking it through, birth is about children . . . and the life and health of our children depend on our actions during (and before) pregnancy. The Bradley Method's goal is to present honest information about a natural process in a simplified way.

The doctors talk about the benefit/risk ratio when evaluating the usefulness of medical procedures. I prefer the term "choices". I feel that the reason God gave children parents is so that someone who cares and has a continuing responsibility will make the choices. Parenting is, perhaps, life's greatest experience. Parents (and their babies) must live with, and often pay for, the choices they make.

Natural childbirth is the standard . . . all interventions must be weighed against this standard. In obstetrics, procedures are often measured against what is routine, not what is natural.

As parents, we have been living with the results — psychologically and

---

Many of the things I will talk about in this chapter may be lifesaving in specific circumstances or of great benefit once in a while. Labors should be evaluated on an individual basis, not routine. Machines cannot replace good personal care. Nothing in this chapter is meant to be a criticism of any particular individual, but rather is meant to inform consumers about risks which do or may exist.

physically — of the choices WE made. At times we made choices we didn't even know we were making. When you choose a physician, for example, you are not only choosing a person whose personality you find compatible, but you also (often unknowingly) choose the prejudices and routines that were a part of his medical training. When you choose a location for your upcoming birth, you choose between the risks and safety of home, birth center, and hospital. And make no mistake about it . . . EACH choice has its own risks, as well as benefits, as does almost everything you do in life.

In the next few pages, I'll try to share with you some of the things I've been able to learn about birth. The main point I'd like to leave you with is this . . . GOD GAVE YOU THIS BABY . . . TO LOVE AND CARE FOR . . . YOU MUST MAKE THE CHOICES YOURSELF . . . NOBODY CAN DO IT FOR YOU . . . YOU MAY MAKE THE WRONG CHOICE, BUT ONLY YOU CAN CHOOSE . . . BEAR IN MIND THAT YOUR LIFE, AND YOUR BABY'S LIFE IS AT STAKE . . . PLEASE . . . DON'T BELIEVE A WORD I SAY . . . OR ANYBODY ELSE SAYS . . . YOU MUST LEARN, PREPARE, HIRE AND FIRE, STUDY . . . AND CHOOSE!

I'll try to go over the risks and benefits of many of the choices you must face when you are pregnant . . . remember I am a biased, prejudiced person . . . in many cases I select those studies that support MY prejudices. It is important that you know, however, that **your** doctor, like all doctors, may be a biased, prejudiced person also, selecting (or in more cases than not, being selected for) those studies that his school or his detail man (drug salesman) call to his attention. As David Stewart has pointed out . . . 'TRUTH IS NOT DETERMINED BY MAJORITY VOTE.' All the obstetrical, governmental, psychiatric committees on earth cannot change the truth. They merely control the behavior of those who submit to their authority. You do not have to submit. You CONTROL them. You hire and fire doctors and hospitals, midwives and other personnel. The Doctors have given up much of their control to committee vote. If they disagree, they dare not tell the patient (their privileges are at stake). If a nurse disobeys the rules, she may be fired. The only person free of the rules, laws, and 'routines' is you — the parent. Know your rights! And, exercise them!

Since common sense and 'natural processes' are so frowned upon in our pseudo-scientific world today, I will try to include references to the medical literature so that medically-oriented folk can look them up. But, again, remember . . . for each reference I chose, there are often others, also done by competent, sincere researchers whose conclusions may be much different. Indeed, many of the authors I shall cite, drew different conclusions . . . again YOU must decide.

The natural birth process works well in most cases. Any deviation from nature should rightly be considered **dangerous** until **proven** safe!!

We live in a world WE consider "modern," but our great-great grandparents **thought** they did, too! Our great grandchildren will judge us harshly for our ignorance of natural birth!

The normal process of birth remains the same, but today's procedures harm far fewer than did Dr. Semmelweiss' peers (who often killed 20 to 30 percent of the mothers they were 'helping'). At Boston Lying-In Hospital in 1883, 75 percent of the mothers had childbed fever, and 20 percent died of it. In 20 years we may look back at today's practices with the same disdain that we, today, reserve for leeches, and bloodletting. But, remember, THEY WERE MODERN in their day!

66

BIRTH LOCATION

This is, of course, one of the key decisions on which many of the others hang. In today's world "the hospital" has been the typical birth location for most American births (deliveries) and has pros and cons.

For many, the hospital symbolizes sterility, competence, medical "safety" and peace-of-mind. Many hospitals have now, in effect, realized the absurdity of their past practices . . . they now "admit" or "allow" fathers at birth. Remember, every time a medical "sacred cow" fades into obscurity (silently, of course) that this **in itself** is evidence of the fallibility of the present system. THE DOCTOR WAS WRONG! Most of the same people who now embrace "fathers in delivery" as their own invention, have never given credit, or so much as a "thank you" to Robert A. Bradley, M.D., who first conceived the idea of the husband as an active, participating labor coach over 30 years ago.[1] Most of these self-appointed barricaders of delivery rooms would have said (and many did) only a couple of years ago that husbands were either (a) unnecessary, (b) dirty, (c) lawsuit-happy, (d) crazy — or often all of these and more. I'll bet your local hospital has changed its policy toward husbands since 1970 or later. Ask them. I bet they won't want to tell you. Dr. Bradley was called every name in the book, (and sometimes still is) and every dirty trick you can think of was thrown into the battle — but THEY LOST — CONSUMERS (PARENTS) won the war.

Many people, in fact most people today, choose to give birth in a hospital. Dr. Bradley insists, "Make the hospital more home-like."

Many hospitals today are opening "birth centers" in the hospital where uncomplicated births can be carried out in a "pseudo-home" but with all medical personnel and equipment available — fast. Many of these hospitals are making real "progress" toward a more natural birth environment.

A word of caution . . . because the public is becoming more aware, many hospitals have begun to give lip-service to the "birth center" concept. Changing the signs, or answering the phone "birth center" does not make it one. Many hospitals today promote "family-centered maternity care" without even understanding the words. Many hospitals offer a "Leboyer" birth, and all that has changed is that after the labor is stimulated, the mother is drugged, the baby dragged out, the routine episiotomy is performed, and all the insanity of "delivering the baby" takes place. Then, the "poor kid" is dunked for a few seconds into a plastic bathtub — and all concerned are placated — at least all but the poor child. There are now many birth centers, but very few UCCs (**un**medicated childbirth centers). BEWARE OF THE BAND-AID APPROACH!

So, the pros of the hospital are peace of mind (very real to some people) and the availability of medical intervention. Ironically, the hazards of the hospital may be exactly the same — very real fear of the hospital (just as real to other people) and the risk of unnecessary or botched-up medical intervention. Dr. Robert Mendelsohn states,[2] "People who say the hospital is the only safe place to have a baby just don't know anything about hospitals." He goes on to state the hospital has three categories of risk: (1) bacteriologic, (2) psychologic, (3) accidents. To these you must add the increased risk of intervention — if the machine is there, why not use it? There are whole new strains of germs that exist ONLY in hospitals, and the rate of infection is much higher in hospitals than at home (four times as high!)[3]

The out-of-hospital birth center is also gaining in popularity. The NACHIS Birth Center in Los Angeles is an example of a birth center in the doctor's office. Vic and Salee Berman have structured their OB practice around natural childbirth and achieve over 90 percent unmedicated, spontaneous births.[4] (Of their first 109 attempted birth center births, 101 were successful; eight were delivered in the hospital and only one needed a Cesarean section). It was a good idea to ASK what is your doctor AND hospital's rate of medication, forceps or Cesarean section BEFORE selecting them!

The pros of the birth centers are the freedom from many of the routines and rigid practices of the past . . . often coupled with truly personal care. The cons are the removal of the pregnant person to another place, and the collecting of these people in a central location for the convenience of the personnel involved. Also, I suspect that the rate of infection will be shown to be much lower than the average hospital, but not quite as low as the home. The pregnant couple and their unborn baby have already been exposed to the bacteriological environment of their own home. When a large number of people are collected in one place — some are sick or contaminated — the risk of spreading an infection is much higher.

The care which the pregnant person receives is generally undivided in her own home, semi-divided in the birth center, and almost totally impersonal in most hospitals where everyone works by the clock and shift changes turn the entire institution over to a new crew at one time. As the home and birth center become more popular, they, too, run the risk of becoming impersonal — a doctor or midwife with two, three, four people in labor is in a real bind. The tendency to "hurry" labor is very hard to resist. This can leave the staff without options and lead to a rushed . . . assembly line. Birth is a slow, individual process, to be savored and enjoyed slowly. The safety of the process is MOST THREATENED BY RUSHING MOTHER NATURE.

Home birth is also making a strong comeback. Gregory White, M.D., author of "Emergency Childbirth" has stated "home birth, in properly selected patients, properly attended, is as safe as hospital delivery — I have a hunch they may even be a little safer. If I didn't think so, I wouldn't be doing them!"[5] At NAPSAC, after presenting a matched study of 1046 home/1046 hospital births, Dr. Lewis Mehl concluded,[6] "Compared with birth in the home, 3.7 times as many babies required resuscitation; infection rates of the newborn were four times higher; and there were over 30 times more birth injuries in the hospital. As for the mother, in the hospital there were 2.5 times more oxytocic stimulants used during labor, 22 times more use of forceps, nine times as many episiotomies (which are supposed to prevent tearing of the perineum). Yet, there were nine times as many severe lacerations as in the home."

Almost everyone who received the interventions in the hospital were made to believe that the hospital "saved them." The only way to truly make the hospital more home-like involves retraining the mistrained, not changing the signs.

BIRTH ATTENDANT

The second point is the choice of the person to attend the birth — doctor (either obstetrician or general family practice) or CNM (certified nurse-midwife), or lay midwife, or other medical or para-medical person. There also exists a growing number of families who opt for NO attendant — the DIY (do-it-yourself) birth.

Again, the pros and cons...

The doctor ... a few doctors are specializing in births — while the mainstream of the profession prefers "obstetrical management" and "deliveries." Be sure you have chosen the type you wish. If you want a hospital birth ... many fine doctors will be happy to perform "life-guard" duty and merely "catch" your baby if all is well. But, also there are the other type who "always" need to use IVs, fetal monitors, forceps and the like. You might ask your doctor what is HIS rate of Cesareans, forceps, and episiotomies? Also "Do you KNOW HOW to deliver a breech baby?" or "Do you KNOW HOW to do a pressure episiotomy?" Did you know that the word "physician" comes from the Greek word for "natural?"

One more thing about doctors — if your doctor doesn't do home births, don't try to 'twist his arm'. The skill that most doctors learn for deliveries is simply not safe for use at home birth. If your doctor hasn't done home births, but wants to learn, there are two groups which may help him learn.[7]

About midwives, the American College of Nurse-Midwifery has generally been anti-home birth in recent years. Many CNMs (certified nurse midwives) are not trained in home birth. Many of the midwives around the country who are lay/professional/licensed are totally untrained. Many others are self trained and may be very skilled. Again, only you can choose.[8]

The choice to have a midwife is increasing. The number of self-taught midwives has suddenly become a major factor in the choices available. A word of caution: what training there is for midwives has most often been along the lines of the physician training. In many big city hospitals the midwife does the same things the doctor did — only the midwife has LESS freedom to vary "routine" to fit the labor. The assumption that a slow labor is "bad" and a fast labor is "good" still rules! The idea that second stage labor should last only a few minutes is dangerous. Routine episiotomy and other interventions, once voted in, are often mindlessly carried out by personnel too "chicken" to be different.

A word about the feminist movement. Lately there is an assumption that FEMALE attendants are naturally better than male — that all women are sisters, and only a woman can empathize with another woman. Maybe this is right but I doubt it. Cast your mind back over the history of childbirth — Dick-Read, Lamaze, Bradley, Brewer, DeLee, Semmelweiss, Leboyer — all were males. These MEN have contributed greatly, not only to the technological safety of birth, but also to the feelings, joy, pride of the MOTHER, the FATHER.

Today we have many concerned females — and more power to them — but also we have unconcerned, sadistic and political women. It is NOT SEX that determines human-ness ... and neither sex has a monopoly!

P.S. I don't mean to diminish the contributions of the female pioneers who have taken more than their share of punishment, trying to help us all. A couple of names many of you will never be able to thank enough are Charlotte Aiken, Margaret Gamper, Mabel Fitzhugh, Doris Haire, Rhondda Hartman, Carolyn Rawlins, Beatrice Tucker, Marjorie Karmel, Lynn Moen and seven ladies from Franklin Park who changed the entire western world. Without them the rest of us might never have learned what we were missing.

A word about DIYs (Do-It-Yourself) ... in this book you will see pictures of the

Stewart family's latest birth (Anthony) and other kids — each, a DIY — helping. Lee Stewart, writing in "21st Century Obstetrics" explained their decision...

"Fourteen years ago we had to make our choice — our choice of how our baby would be born, a choice about how to feed our baby, a choice about a way to raise our baby that was best for him. At that time the so-called scientific evidence did not agree with our own strong feelings and common sense.[9]"

David wrote, in "Safe Alternatives in Childbirth," "It is usually the parents who are the most informed and who care the most for the safety of their baby who choose a home birth. Those who are least informed usually relinquish themselves to doctors and hospitals without question."[10]

In a medically unattended birth there exists a small possibility (but very real) that some medical emergency could occur and that treatment would be delayed enough to kill somebody. In a medically-attended "managed birth" the risk may be that a normal, healthy mother or baby may be killed because of intervention. I, personally, am unsure which is the **greater** risk. Dr. John Bonica, author of "Obstetric Analgesia and Anesthesia" spoke at the ICEA convention in Seattle in 1976. He shouted to the audience "all anesthetic deaths are preventable." He may be right. But, unfortunately all anesthetic deaths are not prevented.

So, choose the attendant with care, and skepticism. Even the best can make a mistake. Be sure YOU have as much control as possible — not the other way around. Also, take into account their number of patients — a totally exhausted birth attendant MAY make mistakes, or hurry an otherwise natural labor.

DRUGS IN PREGNANCY

The American Academy of Pediatrics Committee on Drugs has stated that there is no drug which has been proven safe for the unborn child.[11] If that isn't strong enough, recall the DES tragedy that we are now living through, or the Thalidomide tragedy a couple of years ago. In both cases the drugs involved were thought to be SAFE! In the American Journal of Obstetrics and Gynecology, December 1952, page 2, a full page ad told your doctor "...DES RECORDS THE HIGHEST RATE OF FETAL SALVAGE ... NOW AVAILABLE NEW DES POTENCIES FOR MASSIVE DOSAGE THERAPY." Today these children have been told the risk of certain kinds of cancer threatens them and they live under a cloud.[12] In November of 1971, almost 20 years later, the FDA Drug Bulletin contra-indicated DES is Pregnancy.

This illustrates the basic thesis of the Bradley Method, "It's not NICE to fool Mother Nature!" In medicine, everything starts out SAFE, then all too often is QUIETLY withdrawn later. We are all "experimental animals" in the overall scheme of medicine.

The average woman during pregnancy takes 10.3 different drugs; 97 percent of the women take prescribed drugs, 65 percent self dosed.[13] — all of them an **unknown** threat to the unborn baby. The medical establishment and the March of Dimes often say, "Don't take any drug ... unless it is prescribed by a doctor!" Since the doctor has absolutely no way to know if **ANY** drug is **SAFE,** what a useless piece of advice this is. The doctors of America are the biggest drug-abusers of all time, according to Robert Blake. TV's Baretta. "78 percent of American suicides are committed with prescription drugs... The doctors give out more dope than the junkies!"[14]

NATURAL VS. UN-NATURAL BIRTH

How often have you heard the phrase, "Oh, I could never go natural" or "Don't be a martyr . . . a little relaxer won't hurt" or "I'm a chicken . . . knock me out . . deliver the baby . . . send me to the hairdresser, and then wake me up."

Quite apart from the medical risks of un-natural childbirth is the psychological hazard. The basic drive that people have to reproduce is not a new thing. The basic function of any species is to reproduce itself. Planned (un) Parenthood and ZPG not withstanding.

Ask yourself why so much emphasis on "Don't feel guilty if you. . . " In spite of all the platitudes on earth, if you have certain goals and can't fulfill your own expectations, you will have a problem. This is true regardless of the process involved. If you set out to win a race, and lose, all the sympathy in the world doesn't compensate fully, right?

The birth process **is** an athletic contest of sorts. Elizabeth Bing, co-founder of ASPO states "I know you'll be happy to hear that we don't intend to make martyrs of you or even athletes. We certainly believe that medication can be helpful."[15] This, if I may be partisan for a moment, is the basic difference between Bradley and Lamaze. In JOGN Nursing, March 1977, a spokesperson for ASPO stated "the description 'prepared childbirth' is more appropriate to Lamaze than 'natural' — a term that is more often associated with Bradley." Seven paragraphs are offered titled "Lamaze vs. Natural Childbirth." For years the Lamaze groups have said "we are not natural childbirth." I, for one, believe them.

I think it is important for the family in a multitude of ways to have a NATURAL birth. All the talk of guilt is interesting. Could it be that there is something important about the birth process that is SO important that those who participate in its repeal are so "hung-up" with guilt.

Dr. Bradley maintained 96.4 percent of natural births in his first 8000 births.[16] The process seems to work doesn't it? In Montevideo, Uruguay, Dr. Roberto Caldeyro-Barcia IN A HIGH RISK REFERRAL CENTER maintains 90 percent.[17] The American Academy of Husband-Coached Childbirth has teachers all over the country who maintain 80 to 95 percent unmedicated births, year after year. THE PROCESS WORKS!

Prepared childbirth has often meant just what it says. You get prepared for what is routine. You have to set goals for yourself, become motivated. No outside person can do this for you. If you set high standards for yourself and your baby, I believe you can expect to reach your goal over 90 percent of the time. If you set low goals, you can bet that the chance of attaining anything is also low.

Guilt is a word we hear a lot about today. We are told that "if it feels good, do it;" that marriage, families, chastity, fidelity are "old-fashioned!" We are told over and over not to feel guilty. Could it be because those who are telling us not to, are? We are told that a mother in labor "shouldn't be a martyr." I wonder how many would listen to the same advice if you knew your child was in danger — suppose your young child was playing in the path of a freight train — suppose there was one chance in 10 that you could get to the child in time — suppose you might be killed yourself. Would the same do-gooders tell you not to be "silly." What more important cause is there to be a martyr for?

SOME SPECIFIC ISSUES

RELAXER

Obstetrical analgesia (relief of pain) is relatively new, relatively dangerous, and even relatively INEFFECTIVE. Many mothers report that when they were given narcotics they experienced MORE pain, but because they were quieter, they were thought to be getting "relief." The attendants often confuse "quiet" with "comfort!"

Calling a narcotic drug or narcotic potentiating drug a relaxer most certainly is malpractice, in and of itself. Heroin is heroin — and so is demerol (almost). A narcotic is a narcotic and changing the name doesn't help.

The ill effects of drugs of the baby were noted as early as 1885,[18] but most doctors want us to think they were just discovered! The average doctor, a couple of years ago, talked reverently about the "placental barrier," only one of the myths to disappear under the light of consumerism. Fox[18] reports "the fetus today CONTINUES to be the INVOLUNTARY recipient of (analgesic) agents, "ALL analgesic agents administered to the mother are capable of reaching and AFFECTING the fetus. The clinician should resist the temptation of premature and perhaps unfounded self-congratulation when an infant, not affected by these gross measures, is born to a medicated mother."

All narcotics (demerol, morphine, heroin, meperidine, nisentil, talwin, mepergan, etc.) transverse the placenta to the fetus and all exert direct central nervous system DEPRESSION on the fetus of the newborn."

Doris Haire said it well. "Many professionals contend that a 'good experience' for the mother is of paramount importance in childbearing. They tend to forget that, for the vast majority of mothers, a healthy undamaged baby is the far more important objective of childbirth. The two objectives are not always compatible. Human maternal response has not been demonstrated to be adversely altered by a stressful, unmedicated labor if the mother has been prepared for the experience of birth. To expose the mother to the possibility of a lifetime of heartache or anguish in order to insure her a few hours of comfort is a misguided kindness."[19]

T. Berry Brazelton, writing in "Redbook Magazine" says "In our medicated society we have eradicated some of the pain and anxiety but I'm afraid we have eradicated more of the excitement and joy!"[20]

As far as narcotics go, I think that's enough. As for the tranquillizers that sometimes are used with narcotics — "VALIUM IS CONTRAINDICATED IN INFANTS"[21] — need I say more!

X-RAY

Remember when X-rays were SAFE? Heck, I even remember when aspirin was safe! Remember the X-ray machines in shoe stores? Why, X-rays were so safe they even treated sore throats with them, remember. Well, a good friend of mine remembers. She had a sore throat when she was a kid — might have been her tonsils. Today, many years later, she has a **real** sore throat. She had thyroid cancer surgery just last week. Like I said, it WAS safe!

ULTRASOUND

Unlike X-ray, ultrasound is safe?Most American physicians and midwives give radiation from doptones, monitors, and so on, to almost every kid they see — or

72

more precisely, listen to. Many report the mother is "thrilled" to hear her unborn baby's heartbeat! Many feel it is wonderful to be able to hear the heartbeat during labor and to connect it to a machine. Nobody much seems to care that irradiating the baby MAY cause a few side effects. After all, it saves time doesn't it! And it is safe! Or, is it? A couple of the many reported side effects (in laboratory animals, I hasten to point out) are gross cranial and facial malformations, breakdown of DNA molecules, induced chromosome damage, blood stasis, liver cell changes (jaundice?), reduction of antibodies. Well, you get the idea.[22]

At NAPSAC Doris Haire reported a Dr. Susuki of Japan expressed concern over the ovum of the unborn sonnicated female children — might they be rendered sterile? Doris asked, "Will ultrasound be the DES of the next generation?"[23]

Ultrasound scanning techniques scan ultrasound energy through (or at) every centimeter of the unborn, insuring total exposure. This produces a visible record of the relationship of the child to the placenta and the mother's pelvis. In external fetal monitors, the sonar radiation may be continuous (rather than pulsed) and may bombard the infant for hours, or even days.

AMNIOCENTESIS

This is passing a needle through the mother's abdominal wall and into the uterus, withdrawing a sample of amniotic fluid for laboratory analysis. There are three major categories of risk. Fred Ettner, M.D.,[24] has reported on the risks of the procedure itself. It might be safe unless the baby is punctured (eye, scrotum, umbilical cord); the fluid leaks into the mother (peritonitis); the baby's and mother's blood mix (rh sensitization); the placenta is punctured which may lead to abruptio placenta (premature separation); or perhaps, fetal exsanguination (the poor kid bleeds to death). Is it safe? The parents must choose.

So, the first risk is that the puncturing may not puncture what was supposed to be punctured. To this risk, add the risk that the laboratory may mess up the test leading to a second attempt or a misdiagnosis. Did you know that at U.S. Senate hearings in 1975, reports showed 25 percent (one out of four) medical-laboratory tests performed in the U.S. are substandard or wrong![25] Let us assume that the punctured person survives and the lab doesn't mess up — then, what? We encounter the other two risks. First, the baby seems okay, so the doctor thinks he can schedule the delivery to fit his schedule, or yours, or the hospitals. Second, the baby is not okay. This leads to a large percentage of fetal deaths — abortions — death by doctor. They perform abortions to kill those who don't measure up. In California an obstetrician is on trial at the moment, accused of entering the nursery and strangling-by-the-neck-until-dead, a baby in an incubator whose only crime was to live through a saline abortion. MAY GOD HAVE MERCY!

DIETS VS. DIET

Have you heard Dr. Tom Brewer? If you have, you already know what's coming. If not, you should. Probably no other area of prenatal care has as great a potential for benefiting the unborn as Tom's. The basic choice revolves around the historic (and wrong!) medical advice, i.e.: avoid salt, don't gain more than "X" pounds, take "water pills" (diuretics) or "diet pills" (amphetamines-speed) and other drugs. Don't worry, the baby is a parasite. Only a couple of years ago these were the stock-in-trade of your local baby shrinker.

The subject needs more time and space than we have here. I made a film, "Nutrition in Pregnancy,"[26] with Dr. Brewer, and Tom and Gail have written a great book, "What Every Pregnant Woman Should Know."[27] I recommend both of them to pregnant couples. Many Bradley teachers all over the country have copies of the film.

Briefly, the message is simple. EAT A GOOD, WELL BALANCED DIET, RICH IN PROTEIN, SALT YOUR FOOD TO TASTE, AND AVOID DRUGS. Remember you are, in fact, eating for two. The risks of medical science are nowhere more visible (and TRAGIC) than in the way the average doctor, too busy to evaluate the evidence, bought (hook-line-sinker) the polished, well-financed promotion of the drug industry. Tom calls this Thalidomide II. The FDA has only recently (quietly) held hearings into diuretics at Dr. Brewer's insistence. On July 17, 1975[28] "Certain Thiazides — Their Use in Pregnancy" at which many doctors, Tom among them, tstified about the use of diuretics. One even testified using these dangerous drugs ". . . is like tearing flesh from her bones."[29] Another questioned, "the unscientific manipulation of data which led to the sensational claims of the private drug industry that sodium diuretics are useful." Shanklin, editor-in-chief of the Journal of Reproductive Medicine described the "wrath of the drug industry" which descended on **him** because he refused to accept their advertising.

Funny how wrath descendeth when advertising $$$ are involved and how little mini-wrath has descended because of thousands of MAIMED AND MURDERED BABIES. At these hearings, incidently, the WRATHEES — the drug industry — did not even have one person to stand up and defend the use of these drugs. P.S. in the Federal Register Volume 41 Number 115, June 1976, under the title "Certain Thiazides," the FDA cited nine companies for "Promoting (diuretics) on NO scientific basis." Perhaps reverse-wrath is in order.

Salt your food to taste. Sound radical? Margaret Robinson in 1958 published a paper in "The Lancet" called "Salt in Pregnancy" in which she compared two groups of pregnant women. Each group has about 1000 women — one group had the traditional "low salt" diet; the other group got lots of salt, even salt tablets!

In the **low** salt group, there was more swelling, more toxemia, and most tragic of all, twice as many babies died!

Your doctor would never use this dangerous routine — would he? Probably not this year, but ALMOST ALL OF THEM DID two, three, four years ago. Funny, do you really suppose that diuretics are street-drugs. Where in the hell DID TWO MILLION pregnant people a year get them if not from the doctor? P.S. if you think you may be a victim of Thalidomide II, contact the SPUN Litigation Center.[29a]

"Nothing is known, Tom's favorite quote from the establishment, is nonsense. In 1941 Winslow Tompkins published a controlled nutrition study — results? Control Group/Nutrition Group — pre-eclampsia 59 to ZERO; Eclampsia five to ZERO; prematures 37 to ZERO. Infant mortality 54.6/1000 to 4.0/1000. This was published in 1941 and many, many, many similar studies since then. If you look at the data one way, a good diet could have saved 50 babies out of 1000. If you look at the same data with a different point of view — something or someone

KILLED 50 babies/1000. Each of these kids was a human being. Each had parents. Each could have been president of the United States, or whatever. It's hard to be unemotional, isn't it?

JUNK

This section has two meanings — junk food and junk junk. To begin, junk food is a recent catch-phrase — but in pregnancy, food is critical. Pure is a word that, in the past, denoted something good. Today when you hear the word, think twice. Pure sugar is an over-refined substance that is actually an anti-nutrient. Pure white flour is flour with all the neat goodies taken out. Low-fat milk merely means that the valuable ($$$) part of the milk is gone — more profit for the dairy. Remember when a high butterfat cow was the prize animal? She still is, only you get the leftovers. Food additives are an area under increasing pressure — finally!

Smoking and alcohol are major threats to your baby. Surprise! Surprise! Remember when three out of four doctors smoked Camels? Remember men on TV with white coats and stethoscopes telling (selling) the ADVANTAGES of smoking? If you smoke, try to stop — or cut WAY down. It is hard, but if you only knew how much it hurts your baby. Also, if you do smoke, eat an even better diet than a non-smoker. This may help compensate a bit!

If you drink a little, why not wait until after the baby is born. Many books told the benefits of a "little drink" for the pregnant "child-woman." You remember how the medical profession talked down to parents as if they were children. It was thought that the pregnant woman is to immature to control herself and should be "controlled" with tranquillizers and alcohol so she could "get through" pregnancy.

Junk is also a term for street (illegal) drugs—heroin, mainly. While there are pregnant women who take heroin, I doubt if they are going to wade this far into **this** book. But, a LOT of pregnant women I have met think they can use a little grass or other drugs. Dr. Bradley says the baby gets about 20 times more of **anything** than the mother (140 lb. mother, 7 lb. baby). In view of this, do you want your baby to get 20 times as high? An adult will most likely decide to postpone these crutches for the sake of the baby. If you could only see and get to know your baby, you would certainly realize the special vulnerability of babies and nothing on earth would induce you to give your baby drugs.

HERBS

Today there is a growing tendency to take drugs in the form of herbal remedies. Many midwives and nature-oriented people believe in certain teas and other remedies. But, remember Dr. Bradley's warning — 20 times more for the baby. If a cup or two of coffee can keep you up at night, what does 20 or 40 cups do to the baby? If a certain tea relaxes you a little, how relaxed is the baby? Remember, many drugs are MORE powerful to the baby than to the mother. There are other, non-chemical treatments for nerves, tension, headache — why not try a nap? Or, a massage? I often hear the argument that if it's herbal, it's natural and it's safe. Garbage! Heroin comes from poppies and we all know how safe it is!

EXERCISE

Rhondda Hartman has written a whole book on the subject.[30] All I can say is — the better physical shape the mother is in for the birth, the better. Birth is a tiring athletic event which calls for the utmost in endurance. Bradley classes all over the country teach the exercises we have found to be helpful. General exercise and overall good health is just as important as specific "childbirth exercises!" A word of caution. I believe, and certain medical authorities seem to show,[31] that lying on your back during pregnancy is a poor idea. I suggest that you find ways to avoid lying on your back as soon as you know you are pregnant.

Dr. Arnold Kegel was an obstetrician who worked with the puboccoxygeous muscle, the vaginal sphincter that surrounds the urethra, vagina, and rectum. An exercise program aimed at this muscle is a great aid to pregnant ladies. If the "kegel" muscle is in good tone before the birth, it is less likely to be damaged or cut during the birth.[32]

ENERGY

Along with the concept of exercise goes the concept of energy. Having a baby is likely to be the hardest work a woman will ever do! So rest is also important. Exercise is not necessarily in conflict with this. Have you ever noticed how much better you sleep after, say, an evening swim? At times you can be emotionally tired, but can't sleep — right? Also, many childbirth methods teach techniques to distract the mother — "funny breathing," (as Dr. Bradley calls it) or "tummy rubbing," or simply keeping your eye muscles fatigued by starring at a focal point, can detract either slightly or drastically from the amount of energy the woman has to deal with her birth. The Lamaze method creates its own "energy crisis" channeling so much energy into distraction. Perhaps this is why Pierre Vellay, the leading spokesman for the Lamaze method internationally, speaking at the ICEA Convention in Anaheim, California, reported with a slide which "demonstrates that if you leave the woman alone, labor will continue for a long time; help her and there is a shorter time — we give medication in 65 percent of cases." His translator, a doctor, very emotionally said "...in the first stage of labor is the woman who goes 10, 12, 20, 36, 52, 72 hours. WE HATE THIS, as ob/gyns. THIS IS HORRIBLE. This is the type of obstetrics we detest completely. We think the ideal method is to shorten the first stage. We like to augment. We like to stimulate. Instead of a first stage 8, 10, 12 hours, WE LIKE TO SHORTEN THAT TIME!"[34] If you teach a method that exhausts the mother artificially, you get an energy crisis.

The fact is that mother nature provides ON THE AVERAGE 12-14 hours of labor. To think that our intellect is superior to nature is absurdity. We have little real idea what labor is all about. The textbooks say first stage is designed to dilate the cervix. This cannot be all that is involved. The cervix can, and sometimes does dilate within a few minutes from say, four to five centimeters to complete. So why the extra 12 hours or so? Is it just barely possible that we have NO IDEA WHAT LABOR IS? By hurrying the dilation we may be short-circuiting other processes that are even more important. Is it possible labor is good for the baby?

ENVIRONMENT

Lately there is a sudden interest in the environment for the birth itself. A French OB, Fredrick Leboyer, has made us all more aware of the feelings and sensitiveness of the new baby.

I feel that we have gone overboard trying to create an abnormal environment for birth. Darkened rooms, hushed mothers, very warm temperature, these are OUR intellectual trips, not nature's. Consider that the baby is not coming from a quiet place, but probably the noisiest place on earth. Consider that the normal chilling of the baby by room air is NATURE'S way to stimulate respiration, and also the normal chilling of the baby may not be a threat (as almost all pediatricians and OBs seem to think). It just may be a response mechanism, not the threat itself. Consider the absurdity of a grown, thinking person cutting off the only source of oxygen (umbilical cord) from a newborn in order to "get the baby to a heater" when nature may be trying to chill the baby to reduce its need for oxygen. Symptomatic medicine often ignores the disease and tries curing the symptoms.

I am not a doctor so I don't speak with authority on matters, medical. I am a photographer and feel I know something about light. The idea that the baby needs a dark room doesn't fit with what I've seen at births. I've seen newborn babies looking at me before they were even completely born. The eye has an iris which adjusts to light. The baby sees in the uterus, or at least reacts to light.

The depth-of-field is a concept in photography which shows that with more light, the iris closes somewhat which makes the area in focus larger. The newborn has no experience seeing at a distance and needs all the help it can get. IT WILL SEE BETTER IN A WELL-LIT ROOM. Just what the baby will see and why it is important we will look at in "BONDING."

One last point, on January 27, 1978 UPI moved a story on the press wires of America warning the hospitals about the use of heaters — radiant warmers often used to bake the newborn. In many hospitals the same kind of fixtures are still in place that heat the french fries at McDonalds. The American Academy of Pediatrics warned more than 13,000 heaters have been sold in the last 10 years. "They are stock items in most delivery rooms." The hazards include first-degree burns, hospital paging systems may interfere with the temperature control, possible cataracts, corneal opacities may result from infrared light. Add to this the very real terror and pain (headache) of being imprisoned under a heater when you can't turnover or shield yourself.

INDUCTION OF LABOR

Artificially beginning labor, usually with oxytocic drugs, is called induction. Augmentation or stimulation is to make an existing labor faster. Many doctors seem to confuse the two. Rarely does an induction stop with induction. Usually the labor is hurried along with additional hormones.

Is oxytocin safe? The Minnesota Maternal Mortality series analyzed 164 maternal deaths. Oxytocin was used in 63 (38 percent). In 25 cases oxytocitics were the direct or contributing cause of death! Sixteen of the 25 were considered preventable![64] I wonder how many of those ladies would today be mothers if they knew what you now know.

However, in spite of the danger of induction, one U.S. hospital announced a few years ago that it will hereafter only be open for OB between 9 and 5. They claim to have a SAFE! method of inducing, and have served notice on Mother Nature — she better cooperate! Absurd, yes . . . but true![35]

The dangers of induction include: The baby may not yet be ready, the mother may not yet be ready, the rate of drugs may be too high, rupturing the uterus, the contractions may be too strong depriving the child of oxygen.

Dr. Bradley has in his book an illustration of an apple tree. Although ALL the apples are the same age, have the same mother, share the same nutriton, they do not all ripen at the same time. The gestation of the human being is variable. Some babies "ripen" in eight to eight-and-one-half months. Others take 10, 11 or more. Neither is sick or in need of medical help — just different. Take your due date and consider it an estimate, at best an educated guess. And for you baby's sake, don't hurry. There are many **pediatricians** who think the "postmature baby" is an over dramatized risk anyway!

If your obstetrician thinks you should be induced, find out why. If you have any doubt, ASK YOUR PEDIATRICIAN FOR A **WRITTEN** CONSULTATION. Most OBs claim total ignorance of the baby after birth; why do we let them make life and death decisions about unborn babies. I think you'll find it hard to find a pediatrician who will PUT IN WRITING, that your baby is ready to be born! Even some of the best guesses — supported by Amniocentesis, ultrasound, X-ray and everything else known to man — HAVE BEEN WRONG BEFORE.

EATING

Hard for some people to believe, but obstetrics has come to believe that, even food itself may be hazardous to your health. At least during labor! This incredible belief comes from the recent "Dark Ages" in OB where almost all mothers were part of what Dr. Bradley calls "Knock-em-Out, Drag-em-Out" obstetrics. In the dimly remembered past — way back when some of **our** older kids were delivered — EVERYBODY GOT GAS. Remember, it WAS safe then.

When a mother has general anesthesia, there is a chance that she will throw up and aspirate (inhale) the stomach contents. This is a medical tragedy that claimed many mothers' lives within the personal experience of most of today's OBs.

However, in the Bradley Method, better than 90 percent can be expected to have a natural birth. If 90 percent of mothers are denied food or drink, you can practically guarantee a larger percentage of Cesareans, forceps, etc.

Now, in very active labor, most women lose most of their appetite anyway and the digestive process seems to slow or stop. Many of the braver birth centers have begun to allow the women TO DECIDE FOR THEMSELVES, if they are hungry or thirsty. Revolutionary, what? Clear liquids or a soft diet may be advantageous.

ENEMA

Nature has provided that early labor is a laxative for most women. This empties the lower part of the bowel making more room for the baby. The "knock-em-out" era brought a host of "routines," each more insulting than the last. This was the last bastion of self-control. No longer could women "be allowed" the privilege of going to the bathroom. They were strapped flat on their back, given an enema and a bed pan, and then cursed at if they messed the linen.

Once in a while the enema stimulates labor and hurries the process. But, why hurry? Also once in a while (often) the enema gets trapped behind the baby's head. This gives the new mother the feeling of terrible constipation along with her contractions. Then, the beauty of birth is accompanied by the screaming of an irritated OB.

SHAVING

One of the other ways the value of womanhood is degraded to the "little girl" syndrome is to shave the pubic hair. When questioned about this absurd practice, most OBs would tell you that it "prevents infection." Have you ever heard that one?

Well, not only does it NOT reduce infection, it actually increases it. Why was it ever begun? The only explanation I've heard is that in the early part of this century the only patients they could get to come to the hospital at all were from the slums — many with lice! So, if YOU have pubic lice maybe then you SHOULD be shaved.

CERVICAL OBSTETRICS (What Is Labor, Anyway?)

Often, the birth attendant judges the progress of labor by the palpitation (touching) of the cervix to determine the "dilation" (opening). Judging the labor by the measurement of the cervix is sort of like measuring an iceberg by the small part above the water!

The cervix is amazingly supple, and any experienced birth attendant can relate many stories of women that have gone from three, four, or five centimeters to complete (10) in a very few minutes. Nature must have had something more in mind than cervical dilation, or else labor would only last a few minutes — but the average labor is around 12 hours — why?

It is possible that the period of labor is very important to the baby and mother for other reasons than just to expel the baby! In Dr. Bradley's practice, even when he knows a woman must have a Cesarean section, he still insists on a period of labor. One reason is to insure that the baby is ready to be born. Often in Cesareans, babies are delivered too soon. (Many doctors have yet to learn they cannot accurately predict the size of the baby and, because they have not yet recognized their lack of understanding of the process, many Cesarean babies are "Iatrogenic" (doctor caused) prematures!

The period of labor prepares both mother and baby for the transition from pregnancy to mother/childhood. Many subtle things are happening during this period. In a few years, as we may begin to see that we don't know enough about the "basics" of labor, someone may begin to produce much of the information that is at this moment unknown.

Some of the possible explanations for this length are: 1) a period of warning — a signal to prepare a safe place and obtain protection; 2) a period of tactile stimulation to prepare the child for extra-uterine life; 3) a period of hormonal adjustment for the mother, to allow time for her physiology to be stable during this tremendous change; 4) a maturation of the lungs and respiratory system for the baby; 5) a period of psychologic preparation. We know now of the unique importance of the first hour **after** birth. What of the labor itself?

It is possible that by scheduling births or by HURRYING them, we endanger mother and child. If a mother has a six-hour second stage, we assume the baby is ready and her uterus is malfunctioning. Is it possible that perhaps the baby is **not** yet ready and nature wants this child to receive extra stimulation in the birth canal. I think this is possible. I have personally observed several births with very long second stages and, in each case the baby appeared to have BENEFITED from the experience although the adults involved suffered confusion and frustration. IT'S NOT NICE TO FOOL MOTHER NATURE.

Our "uterine view" of labor is simplistic, mechanical and dangerous. A slow labor often leads to intervention which often leads to damage. After this kind of cycle, the mother is· told her baby was "saved" and would surely have died. In actual fact, most obstetricians have never ALLOWED a multi-hour second stage. Their theories tell them to hurry. But, they have no idea what harm can come by accelerating the birth.

I have seen babies who were nearly 25 minutes between the birth of the head and the birth of the baby. I have yet to see one of these that appears damaged. Yet, most baby "catchers" feel this is "awful" and some experienced home-birth practitioners brag that they never "allow" over 45 seconds between head and body. What is their rush? The myth of the "fragile fetus" pervades modern obstetrics, and assembly-line hospitals and home-birth attendants have convinced themselves that HURRY is important. Of course, to them time is money — to the baby, he has all the time in the world. The old midwives used to speak of prolonged labor as "a lazy baby." Perhaps they were right.

VAGINAL EXAMS

The over-emphasis on the cervial dilation has given enormous emphasis to the vaginal examination. In the ninteenth century, the "touch" was described. The internal examination of the cervix was performed under drapes. The male doctor is pictured avoiding any eye contact with the genitals or the woman's eyes. In the middle of this century, Ignacz Semmelweiss, a physician in Vienna, discovered and proved scientifically that puerperal sepsis (childbed fever) was an infection introduced into the woman through "the touch."

Curiously, there never seems to have been much discussion about abandoning this fatal practice. In 1883 at Boston-Lying-In Hospital, 75 percent of all mothers had childbed fever and 20 percent died of it![37] The only approach the "scientists" of that century seemed to explore was how to make the examining finger(s) sterile. It seems so simple to merely not do any "touching" but that was not an acceptable approach.

Somehow man's ego just will not allow the birth process remain natural. We are always trying to improve nature. It is important for people to realize that it was not birth itself that was causing these staggering numbers of iatrogenic (doctor caused) tragedies. The medical establishment hasn't made birth safer — it has only reduced the number of mothers killed to an acceptable number.

Today the risk of infection is lowered by better technique and, most importantly by penicillin and more effective treatment. Indeed, the infection rate is still staggering in some of our hospitals, but rarely does anyone die anymore — the drugs "save" them.

The biggest risk today of vaginal examines is that our ego-oriented culture teaches "management" of labor. If the labor process is not yet understood, how can anyone say what is abnormal? Today we have "curves" to follow the cervical dilation. Learned birth attendants "manage" labors to attempt to force them all into a mold.

If the cervix stops dilating, the worst is assumed. Labor, it is taught, must be a continuous process. If dilation stops at five or six centimeters and contractions continue, our ignorance of the process leads often to C/sections for "disfunctional labor." We just don't yet understand the process. If a cervix becomes "complete" then the mother is instructed to "push!" Is it possible that in some labors the first and second stages SHOULD be on separate days? Many mothers who have reported pain in the second (pushing) stage of labor will also tell you they had no urge to push, and the doctors told them they HAD to push based on an internal exam. Just what awful thing is supposed to happen if the cervix dilated and the baby is not quickly ejected is never explained. We live in a mechanical, production-line oriented world. If the door is open, use it quick!

Perhaps this mother should have taken a nap. Perhaps the labor process had not yet finished even though the cervix was 10. Where do we get the idea that labor is a manageable process, anyway. The hormones and manipulation that go with this orientation are harmful, dangerous, and VERY painful. Ask any mother who has had them!

Other hazards of the vaginal exam are: They are painful and interfere with relaxation; they may (accidentally?) rupture the membranes; they often cause a woman to lie on her back, depleting the oxygen supply to the baby; they are undignified, degrading and, very possibly, none-of-our-business. If Mother Nature wanted the cervix inspected during labor, it would be on the outside.

IVs

Everyone who has ever seen EMERGENCY, or other TV-MD shows, has been introduced to the IV — D5W, Ringers — the modern-day medicine man has his cure-all. No matter what the complaint — from heart attack to being run over by a freight train — the TV "cure" is an IV.

The use of IV (intravenous) solutions in labor is, of course, a recent development. The theory behind them is that they 1) provide fluids for the mother and baby; 2) provide a route of administration for the unnecessary drugs and hormones that the "managers" think are necessary.

The dangers are that the mother may be deprived of nourishment by giving her the glucose in an IV (which is hardly a balanced diet). She may not even be allowed to sip fluids, guaranteeing an uncomfortable, at-risk mother to be "managed." The second risk may be even greater now that they have their pipeline in place. They may want to "use it " and administer all manner of junk to the pregnant pair.

The third and latest (yet!) risk is that the glucose given in the IV has been shown to make brain damage in animals easier.[52] The natural process provides that the serum glucose goes down as labor becomes longer than average (not than normal). The "manager" wants to keep this level high! The higher the level of glucose, the greater the infant's demand of oxygen and the sooner brain-damage occurs.

Also, the electrolyte balance of the blood and body are disturbed by fluids and salt in the solutions. We have no idea what the natural body chemistry is. We should not "manage" it.

FETAL MONITORS

The electronic fetal monitor is an experimental device — the "manager's" dream come true . . . the perfect tool . . . the means to remove the business of obstetrics from the realm of midwivery and cloak the profession with the "aura of science!" One of the published benefits of this machine is that it has helped fill the obstetrical residencies of U.S. medical schools.

The fetal monitor records, on paper, the infant's heart RATE, and the contractions of the uterus of the mother. The assumption is that the heart rate tells you how the baby is reacting to labor. There is some argument that the FHR (fetal heart rate) may not be a good indicator of the health of the baby in the first place. Within a few years the current fetal monitors may well be replaced by a second generation that monitors the p02 of the baby recorded from an electrode glued to the baby's scalp.

External monitors use ultrasound-doppler devices to bombard (irradiate, sonnicate) the baby and determine the FHR. The uterine contractions are sensed by a pressure gauge attached to the mother's abdomen.

Internal fetal monitors measure the FHR by screwing a small electrode into the baby's scalp (buttocks, fontanel, eye, scrotum?), or presenting part. The uterine pressure is recorded by passing a tube INTO the uterus and connecting it to a gauge.

Internal monitors require the membranes to be ruptured (more on the joy of this one later) and present a greatly increased risk of infection. They can also produce a very normal-looking graph after the baby has died. They do produce a more reliable graph and do not require the mother to lie on her back.

External monitors generally require the flat-on-the-back position or, at least, the mother remain immobilized. The external monitor can produce poor graphs and lead to misinterpretation and unnecessary interventions.

The scalp electrodes have caused 4.5 percent scalp abcess in the babies[38] . . . but are generally regarded as "safe." After all, X-rays **were** safe, ultrasound **is** safe? What's an abcess or two compared to a device that triples the rate of Cesarean sections...right?

The biggest fear I have about the machines is not the ultrasound (which may be used for DAYS in long labors) or the risk of infection or puncture. I worry about the excuses this device has made for the "managers" to interfere with labor. The rate of C/sections has tripled almost overnight at many hospitals upon the receipt of their first fetal monitors.

If you have a baby who had any difficulty at all during birth, by all means, get a copy of your medical and monitor record. The medical profession would rather the patients (how long must we remain patient?) never find out the supreme and lower courts have held that YOUR MEDICAL RECORDS BELONG TO YOU.

You can see, right on paper the results of interventions — drugs, hormones, rupture of membranes. All these show up clearly on the record and will form the basis of some dandy lawsuits. If a baby is fine, the doctor gives an epidural anesthetic and the mother's blood pressure falls, is corrected, and the baby "delivered." All of the effects of this "management" will be right there on the paper. I wonder what the jury might decide when confronted by a damaged child and PROOF that the epidural anesthesia created a gross insult?

I have encountered many women whose babies were "saved" by fetal monitors. There were never as many babies at risk, or died in labor, than were "saved" by technology! Often a mother's birth story goes something like this: "I got to the hospital and I was doing just fine. They connected me to this marvelous new machine just in time. Thank God for the machine! It saved my baby! No sooner had they connected me to the machine for a little while than a problem showed up. Without the machine they might not have known in time. My doctor says they lost many babies in the old days because they missed the kind of problem my baby had. They rushed me down the hall and did an emergecy C/section and SAVED my baby."

Have you heard this one or some variation of this story. I have — dozens of times.

In order to connect the mother to the internal fetal monitor, they have to BREAK the bag of waters — if it is still intact. When the bag is broken, the cord may prolapse (fall out) with the water. If the baby has a cord around the neck or any place, it could get squeezed. The cord is put under tremendous pressure by the breaking of the bag. The bag of waters is a protection for the baby.[39] It helps EQUALIZE the pressure of the contractions on the baby. Without this equalization, the baby is placed more at risk. When the monitor is first attached it will probably show a normal pattern for a short time while the pressure builds up and the baby becomes more starved for oxygen. After a time the baby's heart begins to show "decelerations" or "dips" which "indicate a lack of oxygen supply to the fetus."[40] The another Iatrogenic (doctor caused) salvation is at hand. The doctor "saves" the baby. He, of course, bills extra for this service!

Doctor Albert Haverkamp[55] has done a study proving the fetal monitor triples the Cesarean rate with no improvement in infant outcome. Until someone PROVES it safe and effective, the monitor remains an experiment — even if it is universally used. Our babies are the guinea pigs in this global "experiment."

FUNNY BREATHING

No, this is not the type of breathing done by obstetrical clowns! Way back, in the dawn of modern OB care, before Dick-Read — or Lamaze or any of the names we know — respiration, breathing became associated with the birth process. In 1956 Fernand Lamaze, a French obstetrician, published "Painless Childbirth,"[42] an instruction in the Lamaze method largely ignored by those who followed and "borrowed" the Lamaze name.

Dr. Lamaze describes the Lamaze method . . . dating back to Dick-Read and Velvosky and Nicolaiev, basing much of his method on Pavlov, and the theory of conditioned reflexes . . . seeking to create a new reflex he called "the contraction-respiration reflex." His criteria set, as a goal, COMPLETE ABSENCE OF SENSATION.[44]

The "breathing" was described as ". . . DIVERSION away from foci of pain represents an analgesic!"[43] "They help with the oxygenation of the blood."[43] The pregnant lady was instructed to "imagine a burning candle some two feet away. Blow on it to bend the flame without putting it out."[45] No wonder one of his patients said ". . . the obstetrician was the conductor; I was the first violin."

Since Dr. Lamaze's book, others have redefined the "Lamaze method." They have included such respiratory symphonies as the "pant 5 and blow," "pant 4 and blow," "pant 3 and blow," "pant 2 and blow," the famous "pant-pant-blow" and the "pant-pant-blow-blow" sometimes erroneously called the "choo-choo." NO WONDER DOCTOR BRADLEY CALLS THIS FUNNY BREATHING. It looks funny, but . . . it isn't funny at all.

In the fall of 1977 . . . ASPO, the largest (but by no means only) Lamaze organization in the U.S., published a booklet for physicians. In it, the outrageous statement is made: "Studies have shown that hyperventilation of the nonanesthetized woman does not cause hypoxia (lack of oxygen) or acidosis (shift in pH) of the infant. This statement is made with no explanation or justification. The same booklet, however, states that "the couple is aware of the SYMPTOMS as well as preventive measures — the laboring woman will either breathe into her cupped hands or a small paper bag." You tell me, if **they** believe this "sales pitch," how come they use the term "symptom" to describe the effects of hyperventilation? Webster describes symptom as ". . . any condition resulting from a DISEASE. . . ."

Let me tell you of some of the studies that have been published in this area. The prestigious British Medical Journal "THE LANCET" in February of 1966[47] published a paper showing ". . . hyperventilation of the mother with or without supplemental oxygen significantly REDUCES rather than improves the oxygen supply to the fetus." Might this not be called hypoxia? As recently as 1978 a journal published an article in which Dr. Gosta Rooth "cautioned" that "maternal hyperventilation during labor can precipitate fetal respiratory and metabolic acidosis. . ." and ". . . a pH drop in the fetus AT LEAST TWICE that seen in the mother."[48]

In the American Journal of OB/GYN "Hyperventilation . . . is an integral party of Lamaze's technique for painless childbirth . . . causes maternal hypotension and PROFOUND ACIDOSIS in the fetus." [49]

The biochemical arguments against "funny breathing" go on and on. The simplest and most important hazard of this technique is that COMPLETE ABSENCE OF SENSATION . . . SHOULD NOT BE THE GOAL AT ALL!

The woman in labor needs all her energy to give birth. There is no reason to ask her to do anything other than labor. Distraction does reduce pain, but labor is hard work, not trauma. Even if "funny breathing" was safe (which it isn't), it still is UNNECESSARY and, therefore, a hazard!

Today many Lamaze teachers teach a "modified" Lamaze which Dr. Lamaze would hardly recognize. These people have often created their own techniques and CALLED them Lamaze. But, they cling to "breathing" as an important "tool" (whatever that means) and often fails to acknowledge Dr. Bradley as the "Father of Fathers". Although Dr. Lamaze did have fathers at some of his births, the father was an observer. The "Monitrice," a professional labor coach, and the doctor were in charge.

EPISIOTOMY VS. TEARING

Williams Obstetrics describes episiotomy as the most common operation in obstetrics, second to cutting the umbilical cord. Why is this? The episiotomy is a surgical (scissors) cut in the skin between the vagina and the rectum. Williams' lists four reasons[50] for doing this procedure: 1) straight, clean incision vs. ragged laceration; 2) spares the baby's head from being a "battering ram" against the perineum; 3) shortens the second stage of labor; 4) reduces the chance of third degree lacerations (serious tears).

Many doctors believe in episiotomy for **every** birth. Let's examine this and see. First, episiotomy is a useful procedure once in a while, especially if the baby is in distress. However, in a conservative practice for the year 1976 in 300 births, the incidence of episiotomy was two percent.[51] that's quite a difference!

Reason Number 1: Is a straight, clean incision easier to repair, or does it heal better? When is the last time you got a "paper cut." Did it heal fast (mine don't)? Some doctors that do few episiotomies have learned to repair a few tears and have been surprised to find that they are NOT harder to work on if you know how. The skin tears through the weakest part, while scissors cut indiscriminately and the muscle (Kegel) is often cut through, leaving a life-long problem.

Reason Number 2: "Battering Ram Theory". No doctor of medicine could possibly believe that perineal tissue is more of a threat to the baby than the cold, hard, unforgiving steel blades of obstetrical forceps, could they?

Reason Number 3: "Shortens the Second Stage." Undoubtedly true. Where is there any PROOF that the second stage should be shorter? (See Cervical Obstetrics.)

Reason Number 4: "Reduces tears into rectum." The problem with this one is that many doctors see their episiotomies extending into the rectum all the time — one in ten, or so — and they are convinced that tearing was inevitable. They don't (are not trained) to consider that the episiotomy weakened the area and made the tear possible. Many busy natural childbirth doctors go years between such lacerations.

Doctor Herbert Ratner, speaking at NAPSAC, said, "Apparently, God, who could make a tree knew not how to make a perineum." He did okay for chickens, goats, but he really "blew" it with ladies' bottoms.

Routine episiotomy and repair makes about as much sense as repairing the hymen after every intercourse.

FORCEPS

I have already commented on the softness and wonderfulness of forceps. Let me share with you a newspaper report Tom Brewer sent me last week. "XXXX County Coroner XXX XXXXX has ruled the death of an infant as an "OBSTETRICAL MISADVENTURE" among the 102 deaths he investigated in 1977. The infant died about 18 hours after her DELIVERY in XXXX Hospital on October 12, 1976. According to her death certificate the cause of death was listed as acute blunt force from an obstetrical instrument (forceps) resulting in a depressed fracture of the skull and acute brain trauma. In an additional written commentary on the infant's death, XXXX stated that the death was "preventable" and that "physician error in judgment and physician error in technique" had taken place.[53]

POSITION FOR BIRTH

"A more or less upright position was used in antiquity, through the middle ages, and until the mid-eighteenth century" reports study published in Obstetrics and Gynecology in March 1958. More recently Dr. Roberto Caldeyro-Barcia, president of the International Federation of Obstetricians and Gynecologists has stated that next to being hung by the feet in labor, the flat-on-the-back position is the worst for labor.

WHEN WILL THE MEDICAL 'PROFESSION' BEGIN TO CORRECT THE IATROGENIC (DOCTOR CAUSED) PROBLEMS THEY CREATE? How many women have needed Cesarean sections because it was more comfortable for the STAFF to have them on their back? Almost every textbook on OB ever printed warns that if the mother's blood pressure drops — get her off her back. Yet almost every labor in the US is done on the back, and almost all DELIVERIES. In our film "Obstetrical Intervention" Dr. Caldeyro-Barcia showed that the size of the pelvic outlet increases by over 10 percent by squatting. Just imagine how many Cesareans could have been avoided!

AMNIOTOMY

This is the medical term for artificially breaking the bag of waters. It has become so common that almost every woman in this country has had it done. Usually all that was required is the woman be, for sure, in labor. It does speed up labor a little (about 35 minutes) and the known risks have been listed as: 1. Cord could prolapse (come out) with the water; 2. Risk of infection in membranes are ruptured more than 24 hours; 3. Failure to work; 4. Bleeding (mother or baby); 5. Placental separation (caused by sudden reduction in pressure); 6. Embolism (rare, but fatal)[62]

No mention is made of the effect on the baby. The bag of waters acts as an equalizer of pressure on the baby, absorbing and distributing the force of the contractions evenly. Dr. Caldeyro-Barcia has reported the increase of swelling, moulding, hemorrhage, brain damage in children exposed to this procedure.[39]

Also Dr. Mehl has questioned the scientific basis for the "belief" that the time limit between rupture and delivery must be less than 24 hours.[63] In one study, there was no increase in risk until the 4-14 day period was reached.

DELAYING BIRTH

If the doctor is not there, the hospital staff often delays birth by one of two harmful and potentially damaging techniques. First, the mother is told to "pant." We have already looked at the risk of this technique. The baby may be hyperventilated just at the very moment it is most harmful. If you have ever tried to hold your breath longer than someone else as a contest, you know that if you breathe OUT (exhale) you can hold your breath a little longer. This is because the desire to breathe is controlled, not by oxygen, but by CO_2. The hyperventilated baby may not WANT to breathe, even though severely in need of oxygen.

The second technique, believe-it-or-not, is to put the woman's legs together. Often this is done by tying her legs together with the sheet. I know this is hard to believe. Many doctors, of course, would never allow this to be done. But, remember, the doctor is not there. Even though it's hard to believe, I know many babies who got this "treatment".

The president of United Cerebral Palsy warned that holding back babies "is resulting in brain damage."[56]

ANESTHESIA

Unmedicated birth can be painful, but the effects of drugs may cause pain for a lifetime. All anesthetics are dangerous, and it is beyond me why learned doctors can't accept the alternative of no medication. Unless absolutely necessary, drugs are an un-acceptable risk. In a **high-risk** center Dr. Caldeyro-Barcia has reduced the percentage of patients receiving **any** kind of drugs to 10 percent — Dr. Bradley, in his practice has 96.4 percent unmedicated . . . it can be done, anywhere.

CUTTING THE CORD

A controversy exists over the proper time to cut the cord. Those who are in a hurry often cut the cord seconds after birth. The common belief in our society in that the cord cutting is somehow associated with "turning the baby on" and that the on-off switch must be located in the cord.

What do you suppose people did before scissors and plastic clamps? Nature has also taken care of this little detail. In fact, it is not necessary EVER to cut or clamp the cord, but after a couple of days the placenta does get a little 'gamey'. If the cord is left alone, for a while, nature will determine the right amount of the baby's blood to leave in the baby. If cut too soon the blood in the placenta (the baby's blood) is lost. One researcher stated that "Early clamping of the umbilical cord is equivalent to submitting the child to a HEMORRHAGE at birth."[54]

Stripping, or milking, the cord may pose a threat to the baby, just to save time. The textbooks tell us that the cord normally continues to pulsate for three to five minutes after birth. If the baby doesn't begin to breathe immediately, the cord is bringing fresh oxygen. The cord is often cut, even though the baby is not breathing — just to allow the baby to be taken to a heater. One last thing — the cord sometimes pulsates for much longer than the books say. At Ann's birth the cord was still pulsating at 20-45 minutes — be patient. IT'S NOT NICE TO FOOL MOTHER NATURE!

BONDING - NURSERIES - SILVER NITRATE

The first minutes and hours after birth are "special." A sensitive period exists where mother and baby form a lifetime attachment. As Dr. Ratner says, a lifelong bosom friendship. Dr. Bradley calls the nursery a "kid concentration camp." There is something so special about this initial period that everyone in the room becomes involved. At first we noticed more motherly mothers, then more fatherly fathers, and then more brotherly brothers — well, you get the idea.

Nurseries came into obstetrics to deal with the baby when the mother was knocked-out in the knock-em-out drag-em-out days. The mothers had been made so sick they couldn't be trusted with their own babies. Today, we have an epidemic of battered children, delinquent children, broken families. Today, researchers[60] have demonstrated the special quality of the early minutes, and some advocate that "allowing bonding" may reduce the incidence of later problems.

Let's look at this thing in perspective. The "allowing" of bonding will not improve mothers and babies, rather the routines of medicine have CAUSED and IATROGENIC (doctor caused) epidemic of unbonded families. Human beings have an intellect and can sometimes overcome an insult. It is posssible that some mothers, themselves "at risk," have not overcome the separation that hospitals have insisted on? In animal mothers, the baby will be rejected and sometimes killed if the bonding is interfered with.

Another way we are interfering with bonding is with silver nitrate, a caustic solution that most states require the attendant to instill in the baby's eyes. The drops kill any gonorrheal infection in the baby's eyes. Or at least, sometimes it does. One doctor advocated, in the Journal of the American Medical Association,[57] that the mothers be treated and the use of silver nitrate be discontinued. This was because he believed the treatment is ineffective. In many parts of the world, routine silver nitrate is not practiced. It causes a moderate "chemical conjunctivitis" (irritation of the eye) usually lasting up to 72 hours[58] with an incidence reported as high as 100 percent.[59]

What the heck, babies are blind anyway, aren't they? Or are they? Many child-development books report they are, but I don't believe a word of it. Anyone who has been at a NATURAL birth can tell you that the babies often look and follow and focus on them BEFORE they are even completely born. If the parents decide (choose) to have the silver nitrate used, perhaps they could wait for a couple of hours. If the parents decide they don't need the silver nitrate, the doctor or hospital may ask them to sign a simple release 'AMA' (against medical advice) form to protect the doctor or birth attendant.

Would you believe that in Cesarean sections the babies are also "treated" even though they have not even been exposed! Such is the logic of today.

Mother nature has provided, once again, that the new baby will be loved and cared-for by a group of people who attend the birth and form a special bond to the new baby. To miss the joy and wonder of a new person's first minutes is tragic. It's not nice to fool mother nature!

BREAST FEEDING
THE VALUE OF VALUES

Mother, O Mother, come shake out your cloth
Empty the dustpan — poison the moth
Hang out the washing — make up the bed
Sew on a button and butter the bread.
Where is the mother, whose house is so shocking?
She's up in the nursery, blissfully rocking.
Oh I've grown as shiftlesss as Little Boy Blue,
(Lullabye, rockabye, lullabye loo)
Dishes are waiting and bills are past due
(Lullabye, rockabye, lullabye loo)
The shopping's not done and there's nothing for stew
And out in the yard there's a hullaba-loo).
But I'm playing "Kanga and this is my "Roo";
(Lullabye, rockabye, lullabye loo).
The cleaning and scrubbing can wait 'till tomorrow
But children grow up as I've learned to my sorrow.
So quiet down, cobwebs: Dust, go to sleep!
I'm nursing my baby and babies don't keep.
Author Unknown —

Dr. Mendelsohn said, "If breast is best, something else is worse." In this crazy world, it is considered rude to "put-down" anything. I'm sure there must be a place for bottle-feeding, but right now I can't quite think of one. The baby needs its mother and the mother needs the baby — it's that simple. The way to get "maximum benefit" from breastfeeding is to breastfeed exclusively (no solids) for four to six months AT LEAST — and then to continue the nursing for a couple of years (until the BABY decides to wean) — to paraphrase Dr. Mendelsohn. I don't know why everyone has been afraid to tell us (parents) this. I guess they think we can't take it or something. But, that's the truth — and you know about fooling Mother.

The medical hazards to bottle-feeding are so great and so scarey (everything from pneumonia to sudden infant death) that, if there was a profit in breastmilk and colostrum there would immediately be a law passed in every state, **requiring** breastfeeding. Perhaps formulas and bottles should be made prescription items, not available easily so mothers wouldn't be trapped into the "occasional bottle" that inevitably leads to another bottle-fed baby. (Why do you suppose the formula companies suddenly have begun to advocate breast-feeding in their multi-thousand dollar ads???) The "free" starter pack that the hospitals give out (formula, bottles, nipples, etc.) should be seen for what they are — the same as the cigarette machine in the hospital corridor — an invitation to need their services again — soon!

For complete information on the womanly art of breastfeeding, contact your local La Leche League.

THINGS THEY STICK IN OUR KIDS

These include bulb syringes, suction devices, vitamin K injections, circumcision sets, billirubin lights, baby warmers — they got a million of them.

Start with the infant's throat; it is assaulted from the time the mouth appears in the belief that God blew-it again. All that stuff in the baby's mouth has got to be removed. Why? Who knows. Thousands of years before they had rubber hoses and such, the babies didn't seem to need them. Today, if a patient during a heart attack coughs, it is seen to help — but if a baby coughs he is assaulted; he gags and learns that the mouth and throat are places of pain. The natural ingestion process is stopped cold. The cycle continues. The baby must fast for 12-24 hours; then we find a new Iatrogenic (doctor caused) disease. Many babies have suffered hemorrhages due to a lack of Vitamin K that NATURE provided be manufactured in the baby's gut as soon as he nurses. Medicine would rather give him a needle. Of course, every time you puncture the baby, there is an increased risk of infection. I have heard of several babies paralyzed by these shots. Doris Haire stresses that Vitamin K (a coal-tar derivitive) has never been tested for carcinoginocity (cancer-causing potential). Nevertheless your baby will probably be stuck with this one without your even being asked.

The pros and cons of circumcision are many. The ACOG is in favor of them. The Academy of Pediatrics is against — you pick.

Jaundice, a new epidemic, is abroad in the land. Anything that you do to the mother or baby may contribute to jaundice. Vitamin K, drugs, forceps injuries, even birth-control pills two years before, have been implicated in jaundice. For many years we taught childbirth classes, and the babies were sent home from the hospital in a couple of hours. The baby wasn't seen by the pediatrician until the end of one month — surprise — very little jaundice. Today, the babies are being "examined" more frequently. Tests are being run more and more often (and the tests themselves contribute to jaundice). Babies are being placed in hospital nurseries (the worst possible place) and then bombarded by flourescent light; most often the same as the ones in your home. This costs a lot. The risk is unknown, but

89

there may be a problem with the burning of the baby's eyes, skin, and changes in the development.

The truth is, we know very little about birth. There are many questions, but few answers. Could it be that our whole perspective on labor is wrong? Could labor be a child-oriented process, geared to the child's needs, and not a maternal process? COULD THE TIME FOR BIRTH BE DETERMINED BY THE CHILD AND NOT THE CERVIX?

Today's answers will become tomorrow's old wives tales.

There has been too much arrogance mixed into our ignorance. Semmelweiss' peers didn't know they were killing their patients, and that was excusable. They didn't have any knowledge of the germ theory. But the arrogance that led to Semmelweiss' ouster and death was not excusable, and the **arrogance** continues today. Semmelweiss' fellow doctors took nearly 50 years to learn what he tried to teach them. They were so arrogant that they believed that "gentlemen don't have to wash their hands." Today, too many are still unwilling to listen. Dr. Tom Brewer has spent 20 years trying to get the "establishment" to listen. They call him names, and put their heads back in the sand. Someday they will understand, and many of them will have to live the rest of their lives with the guilt that will come with understanding.

Doctor Bradley has won a 30-year battle to get the husband to be where he belonged in the first place. The arrogance of his fellow doctors was classic. Read some of the old arguments against husbands today, and they are laughable. We may never know how many tragic problems could have been avoided if only they had listened.

There are many people, doctors and others out there right now, trying to be heard — will anyone listen? There may be some among you, reading this book, who are angry with me for saying all this. For this, I can only apologize. I never meant to attack any individual, although some take criticism personally. I only feel, as a parent, that the medical profession, as a whole, has failed. Parents must assume direct control over their births, and their bodies. Semmelweiss, himself, gave up the struggle to reach the doctors, and as his last, dying effort, passed out leaflets to the public, warning them not to go to doctors.

I have been accused of "scare tactics" when informing parents of the risks and choices available. We don't want to scare people, do we? If you are really interested in "scare tactics" try telling most of the OBs in your town that you don't want silver nitrate (you are blinding your baby!). Or, the experimental fetal monitor (you are killing your baby!). Or, you want to have a baby at home (you are killing yourself!). These learned persons often become hysterical when confronted by rational questions and requests. The American College of OB/GYN says that "Home Delivery (sic) is **child abuse.**" Now, HOW'S THAT FOR SCARE TACTICS?

Dr. Bresky says that "insecurity leads to inflexible positions in medicine." If your doctor is secure, sincerely rejects scare tactics, you can have a most worthwhile discussion; both of you will learn something. Medical training leads doctors to believe certain things. Lester Hazell calls these "beliefs" rather than "truths." Some of them may be factual, and some may be myths. Examining the "beliefs" may lead all concerned to a better understanding of the process and of each other. As David Stewart says "when science cannot so much as tell a mother exactly when her baby will be born, or what will be the sex of her unborn child, how can we expect science to provide reliable guidance to a mother in the midst of labor? The answer is simple, IT CANNOT!"[40] Statistics from the Gregory White, Mayer Eisenstein practice in Chicago for 1976 covering a total of 300 births give you some idea of what natural childbirth, without unnecessary medical intervention can do — Cesarean rate 2 percent; transfer from home to hospital 4 percent; prematurity 2.5 percent; episiotomy 2 percent; and ALL OF THIS ACCOMPLISHED WITH 50 PERCENT FIRST—TIME MOTHERS.[61]

If your doctor or hospital doesn't have similar statistics, you might consider talking to them. If you meet rational objections, consider them carefully. I may be crazy — right? If you meet hostility and ridicule, then you know what you are up against. With our fourth baby, we had to fly to Denver (from Los Angeles. . . 1000 miles) to get what we wanted. If your community has not got the kind of care you want, just remember, it is your baby — and your CHOICE!

REFERENCES

1. Bradley, R. MD **HUSBAND COACHED-CHILDBIRTH** Harper and Row 1965, 74
2. Mendelsohn, R. Film: **ALTERNATIVE CHILDBIRTH** Hathaway Productions 1977
3. Mehl, L. **21st CENTURY OBSTETRICS, NOW** NAPSAC 1977 Page 199
4. **FETAL ADVOCATE** AAHCC 4-468
5. Film: **ALTERNATIVE CHILDBIRTH** Hathaway Productions 1977
6. Mehl, L **21st CENTURY OBSTETRICS, NOW** NAPSAC 1977 Page 207
7. **American College of Home Obstetrics (ACHO)**, 664 North Michigan Avenue Suite 600, Chicago, ILL 60611 **Association for Perinatal Health Care (APHC)** 2522 Dana Street Berkeley, CA 94704
8. **US NEWS AND WORLD REPORT** February 27, 1977 Page 49
9. **21st CENTURY OBSTETRICS, NOW** NAPSAC 1977 Page 9
10. **SAFE ALTERNATIVES IN CHILDBIRTH** NAPSAC 1976 Page 3
11. Haire, D **SAFE ALTERNATIVES IN CHILDBIRTH** Page 19
12. **OBSTET. & GYNEC.** Volume 40 Number 3
13. Enkin, M **MEDICATIONS USED IN LABOR AND DELIVERY** ICEA 1977
14. Blake, R **DAILY VARIETY** March 4, 1977
15. **J.O.G.N. NURSING** Volume 6 Number 2 Page 54
16. Bradley, R **MEDICAL OPINION AND REVIEW** December 1966
17. Film: **OBSTETRIC INTERVENTION** Hathaway Productions 1976
18. Fox, H **EFFECTS OF MATERNAL ANALGESIA ON NEONATAL MORBIDITY** r-427
19. Haire, D **CULTURAL WARPING OF CHILDBIRTH** ICEA 1972
20. Brazelton, T **REDBOOK MAGAZINE** February 1971
21. **PHYSICIANS DESK REFERENCE** Medical Economics 1975
22. **BIRTH AND THE FAMILY JOURNAL** Volume 3 Number 4 Page 127
23. **21st CENTURY OBSTETRICS, NOW** Volume 2 Page 573
24. **21st CENTURY OBSTETRICS, NOW** Volume 1 Page 156
25. Winchester, J **READERS DIGEST** r-419
26. Film: **NUTRITION IN PREGNANCY** Available from Jay Hathaway Productions 4846 Katherine Avenue, Sherman Oaks, CA 91423
27. Brewer, G & T **WHAT EVERY PREGNANT WOMAN SHOULD KNOW** Random House 1977
28. A complete transcript available from: FDA Bureau of Drugs, 5600 Fishers Lane, Rockville, MD 20852
29. **SPUN REPORTS** August 1975
29A **SPUN LITIGATION CENTER** 17 North Wabash, Chicago, IL 60602
29B. Dufty, W **SUGAR BLUES**
30. Hartman, R **EXERCISES FOR TRUE NATURAL CHILDBIRTH** Harper and Row 1975
31. **SCOPE** Loma Linda University Volume 7 Number 11 r-216
32. Berman, S **Film on PC Muscle** 1978
33. Deutsch, R **THE KEY TO FEMININE RESPONSE IN MARRIAGE** 1968
34. Vellay, P **Presentation at ICEA**, Anaheim
35. **MODERN HOSPITAL** Volume 114 Number 6 Page 35
36. **OBSTET. & GYNEC.** Volume 25 Number 4 Page 509
37. Wetrz, R & D **LYING-IN** Free Press 1977
38. **AM. JOURNAL OBSTET. GYNEC** Volume 8 Page 875-8

39. Calderyo-Barcia, R Film: **OBSTETRICAL INTERVENTION** Hathaway Productions 1976
40. **21st CENTURY OBSTETRICS, NOW** Volume 1 Page 299
41. **21st CENTURY OBSTETRICS, NOW** Volume 2 Page 365
42. Lamaze, F **PAINLESS CHILDBIRTH** Regnery 1956
43. **PAINLESS CHILDBIRTH** Page 71
44. **PAINLESS CHILDBIRTH** Page 188
45. **PAINLESS CHILDBIRTH** Page 126
46. **THE PSYCHOPROPHYLACTIC METHOD OF CHILDBIRTH** ASPO 1977
47. **ADVERSE EFFECTS OF HYPERVENTILATION ON THE FETUS** Lancet Feb. 6, 1966
48. **OB/GYN NEWS** Volume 12 Number 1
49. **Am Jr OB/GYN** Volume 91 Page 76
50. Hellman/Pritchard **WILLIAMS' OBSTETRICS** Fourteenth Edition Page 424
51. **21st CENTURY OBSTETRICS, NOW** Volume 2 Page 365
52. **DOUBT RAISED ON WISDOM OF GIVING GLUCOSE IN LABOR** Ob/Gyn News Volume 11 Number 24 r-355
53. **THE TRIBUNE,** Scranton, PA January 23, 1978
54. **JOURNAL OF THE AMERICAN MEDICAL ASSN** Volume 116 Number 23 Page 2573
55. **INFANT OUTCOME HELD NO DIFFERENT WITH EFM** Ob/Gyn News December 15, 1975 4-422
56. THE NEWS March 27, 1970 4-209
57. **JOURNAL OF THE AMERICAN MEDICAL ASSOCIATION** 104:1468
58. **New England Jr. Med.** Volume 274 Number 13 Page 271
59. **Canad. M. A.** 68:117-119
60. **New England Jr. Med.** Volume 286:460-463 r-404
61. **21st CENTURY OBSTETRICS, NOW** Volume 2 Page 365
62. Garrey et al. **OBSTETRICS ILLUSTRATED** Williams and Wilkins rev 1974
63. **21st CENTURY OSTETRICS, NOW** Volume 1 Page 182
64. **OBSTETRICS & GYNECOLOGY** Volume 18 #6

JAMIE BRAGGINS

Pat and Bill Braggins third birth was at the Berman's Birth Center. They prepared their children by talking to them, and showing them movies about births. The labor was slow and transition was hard. The children played quietly with toys

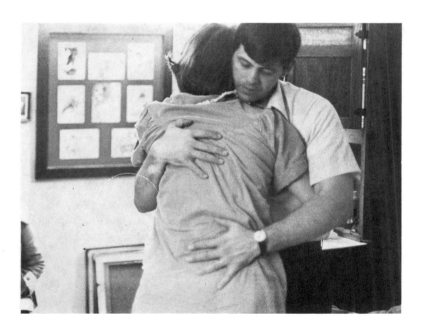

in the reception area of the office. Having friends present was definitely helpful. They were supportive emotionally and physically. They helped with ice chips, juice, cold cloths, rubbing feet and babysitting. The atmosphere was beautiful and serene. All of us missed church for this birth, but Bill said "This is Church!" Each birth renews and enhances my faith in the Lord and assures me of present day miracles.

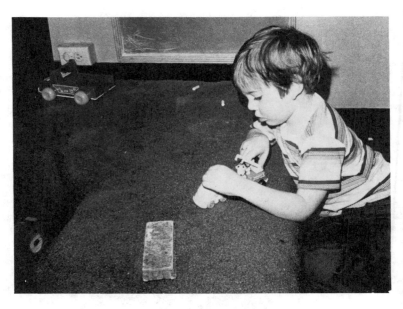

Stephen Braggins (3) Playing During Labor

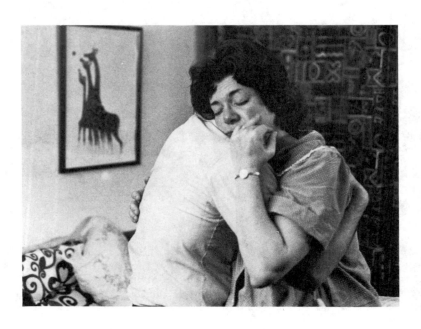

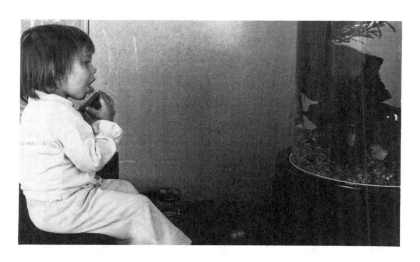

Joanna (1, almost 2) Eats Peanut Butter and Waits

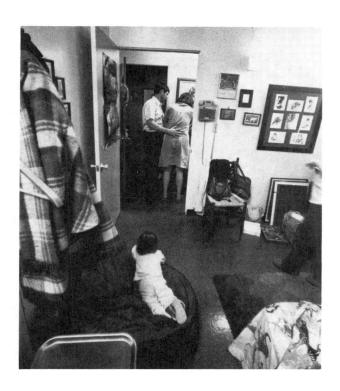

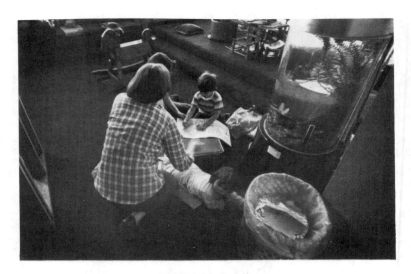

A Friend Babysits

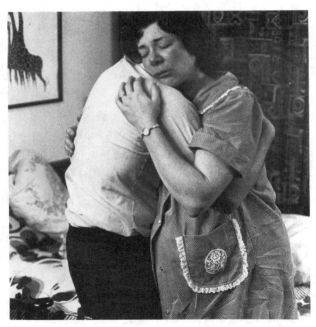

"You've got to coach me and tell me what to do."

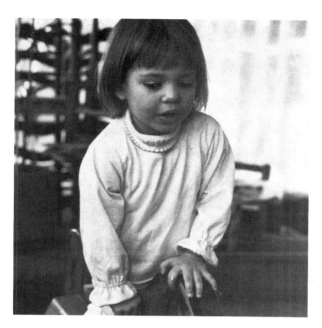

"Push, Baby"

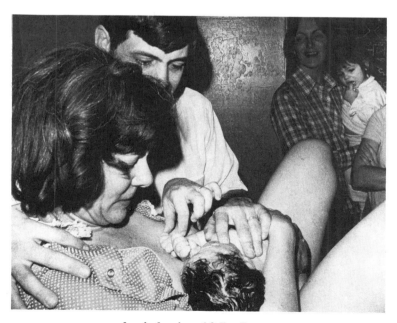

Jamie Louise, 10 lbs 5 oz

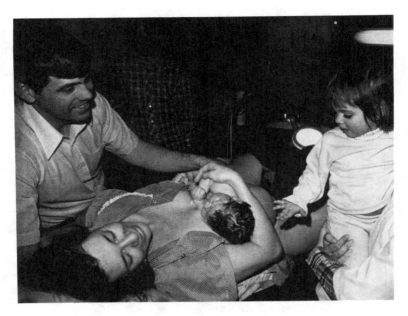

A Real Baby!

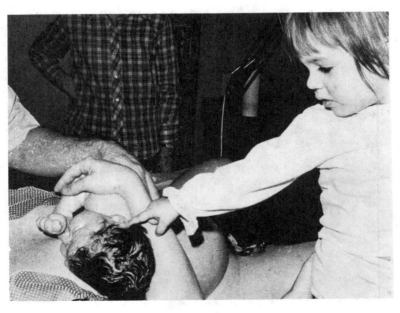

First Touch

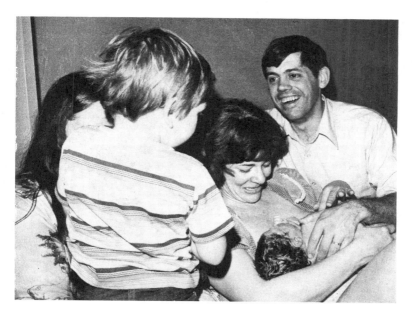

Joy

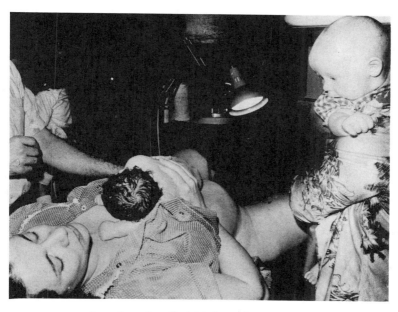

Ann views her first birth, at four months

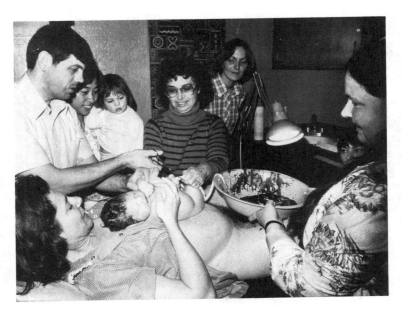

Cutting the Cord After the Placenta Is Out

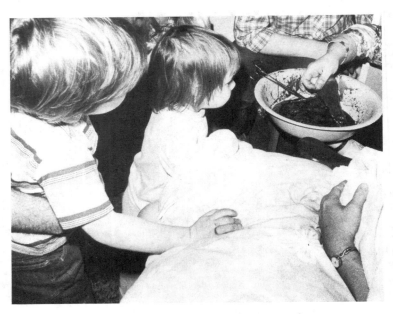

Where Do Babies Really Come From?

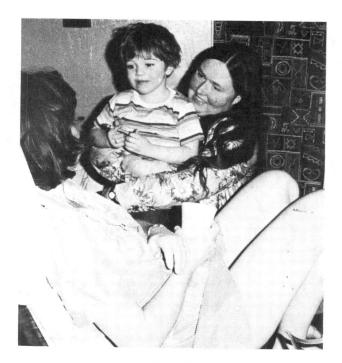

I Love You, Mommy

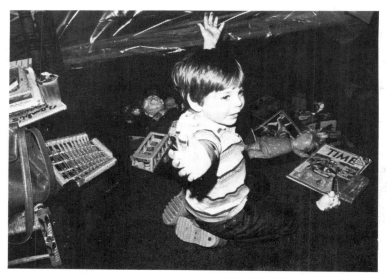

"It's Over, Bye"

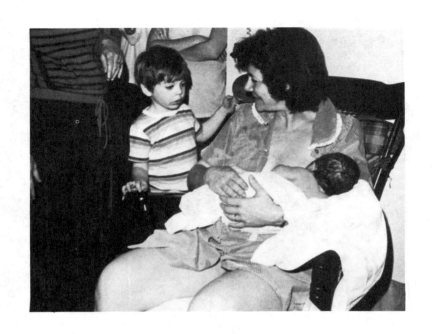

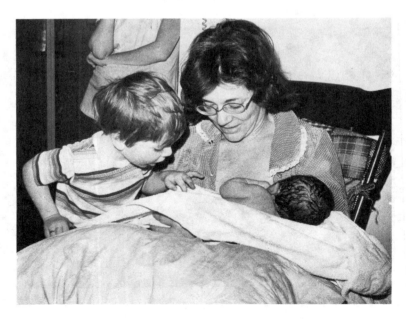

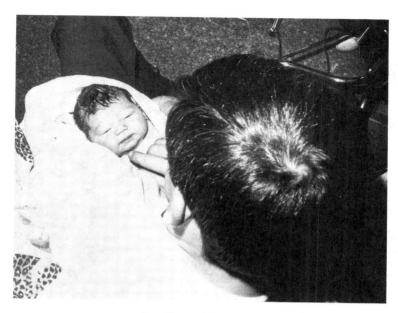

Bonding, with Daddy

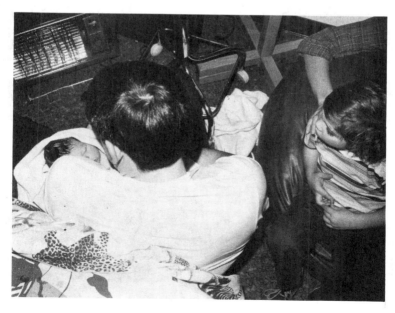

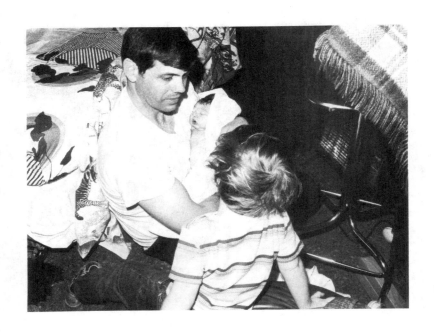

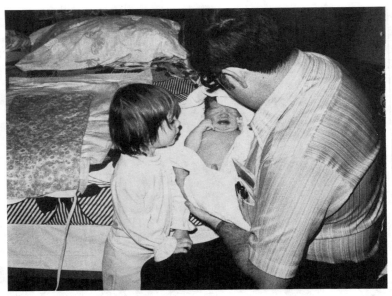

Photographers Also Bond

HOW TO PREPARE YOUR CHILD — SUSAN'S 10 POINTS

By SUSAN HATHAWAY

Perhaps the way to handle most things with children is to keep it simple, honest and natural. Children are able to accept most anything, but on their level. It has been my experience that the same child on different days has different interests. First of all the parents' attitude is important. The attitude should be one of joy and positive expectation. You need to be sure your children have a basic understanding of the facts of birth, but keep it simple.

Our daughter Susan having attended many births wrote 10 points on how to prepare other children for attending births. At the time she wrote this she was 13 years old.

1. Keep in mind that each situation is different. Be prepared to be flexible.
2. The parents must decide if they want the children there first. Then they can be part of the following decisions.
3. Prepare your children:
   a. So they know in reality, what will happen.
   b. Watching childbirth movies helps prepare.
   c. Some kids have said the things that scared them were:
      The baby was blue when it was born.
      The baby didn't cry right away.
      I thought it was too bloody.
   These things should be discussed.
4. Keep things positive.
   a. Avoid medicated birth films. Avoid mechanized medicated birth, because medicated births are out of control and unnatural and frightening. I think it would do more harm than good for a child to be present at a medicated birth.
   b. Parents should be open and willing to talk about birth.
5. Make the children feel important, useful and wanted.
   a. Give them some sort of job to do.
      1) Getting ice chips
      2) Help time contractions
      3) Have them squeeze orange juice
6. Children need a caretaker. Even older children need someone

whose job it is to explain what is happening. This person should be willing to take care of the children if something goes wrong and parents have to leave.

7. Don't neglect other children after the baby is born. They should be part of the bonding process.
8. Don't force anyone especially children to be at a birth.
   a. Some children aren't ready.
   b. Some adults can't take it either.
   c. Depends on their background.
9. You can make a party out of it.
   a. Freeze a cake.
   b. Have orange juice.
   c. Ice Cream.
10. Most of all, please remember that this is a joyful event — a miracle and that whoever is there will remember it for the rest of their lives. So make it as joyful as possible for all concerned.

BIRTH IS FOR BABIES, CHILDREN AND OTHER LOVING BEINGS,

Who See The Wonder and Beauty In Life...

By CHERYL WINES and GLORIA GOOLD

There are few choices that you will make regarding your "birth experience" that will be more important than the careful selection of those in attendance. This freedom of choice is so important. Many couples decide to birth at home largely because that insures that they may retain this right. To say that "the birth experience is affected by the environment in which it takes place," is a gross understatement. Nothing affects the "environment" more than those occupying it. Therefore, the choice of whom to have present at your birth must be given careful consideration. We have seen births at home (and certainly in the hospital), where the experience was far less than satisfactory, **primarily** because of those in attendance. On the other hand, we have observed time and again the eloquent joy expressed and shared by families birthing with those select few that have been **carefully chosen** and **prepared** for the occasion. The key here is obviously **"carefully chosen and prepared."**

Certainly we all have immediate impressions of those with whom we would like to share our births , and those we wouldn't. STOP NOW . . . MAKE A LIST OF EACH PERSON YOU MIGHT CONCEIVABLY INVITE TO THE BIRTH . . . BESIDE EACH NAME JOT A SHORT THOUGHT AS TO WHY YOU HAVE THEM UNDER CONSIDERATION. Now, look carefully at your list:

1. BEWARE of those that you want present **only** because "the experience would be good for **them**"(You want them to see how different it can be")
2. BEWARE of those acquaintances who express an overly enthusiastic desire to attend. Your baby's birth is not a time for "Show and Tell", or to satisfy the curiosity seeker. Exercise your right to say NO!
3. BEWARE of the uninvited guest; the interested party that "came along with so-and-so, just to watch". Exercise your right to say NO!
4. BEWARE of allowing your birth to become a performance,

complete with an audience. Close friends are a comfort, but in large numbers they become a hindrance. We have seen more than one laboring woman whose energies were being usurped by her "friends'" needs. You can find yourselves playing the role of host and hostess at a time when all efforts at comfort should be made in your direction.

5. BEWARE of those people that you can't **truly** "be yourself" with. If ever there was a time when you needed to act and react instinctively, this is it! You probably couldn't do this if you were uncomfortable about what those around you would think.

6. BEWARE of those you feel obligated to (be they birth attendants or close friend). Long after your obligation to them has ceased, your birth experience will be remembered . . . and not by them. This may be the most difficult NO of all, but the choices you make now will remain with you for a lifetime . . . exercise your right.

7. Now, look at your list again and consider . . . do they all WANT TO BE THERE! It is not fair of you to make someone feel obligated to attend anymore than for you to be placed in that position. Unless they truly want to be there, they cannot offer the support and energy you need. It is equally important that they feel comfortable with your birth-at-home choice. They needn't see it as a choice for themselves. However, if they are uncomfortable with it as your choice, then their support and energy will be distorted.

8. The more responsibility you assume for your birth, the more it is not only important, but **vital** to have only those present who truly support you in your birthing choice. Anxiety, fear and various forms of "interference" with birth, can cause havoc with an otherwise peaceful experience. However, BEWARE of inviting an educated or experienced person purely with the thought of relying on **their** education or experience. If this is your desire, then we would suggest that you reconsider the birth choice in favor of more medically-controlled birth. In birth, you must be prepared to accept responsibility, and make choices on your own. Certainly you would regret having invited someone to your birth who "blamed" you for its outcome. If you are secretly relying on someone else to "take care of things," then you are placing an unfair burden on that individual with the possibility of great blame being attached. When you consider inviting someone for "support" be certain you know (and they know) what kind of "support" you're looking for.

Children are often the most joyous participants in the birthing experience. While each child should be carefully considered, the following guidelines 1-7, given the **proper preparation,** they are able to see the birth through the eyes of the innocent; with all of the wonder and beauty that such a miracle deserves. How better to introduce the mysteries of life to a child than by unveiling that mystery to show the simplicity of nature? How better to welcome a brother or sister into the family than as a family? The only necessity at having a child present is that he be well prepared, and that you be honest in that preparation.

Who should attend? Remember, birth is for babies, children and other loving beings who see the wonder and beauty of life. Now that your list is complete, you can issue the "party invitations." Perhaps you should make the provision that when labor actually begins, you may decide not to have others in attendance as many couples prefer not to have company while in labor.

PREPARING PARTICIPANTS
(A Place For Everybody & Everybody In His Place)

The people involved, having been carefully selected, must now be carefully prepared in the role **you** have chosen for them for your birth.

Ways To Prepare

1. Hold at least one meeting with everyone together who will be at your birth. Two meetings is even better. In fact, a weekend where everyone works in preparation for the baby is ideal (making cake, preparing and freezing dinners, cleaning and getting ready the birth area, and so on.) Each person can become comfortable with your home, where things are kept, and feel more a part of the experience.

2. Adults with jobs should be given a list of things you feel important for them to know.

3. Everyone should understand the flexibility of **plans** and know how to back off and not remain rigid.

Things To Keep In Mind For Specific People

1. **Children** can be a tremendous asset at birth. They probably need the least amount of preparation because of their innocent acceptance of anything natural. Be sure, however, you have explained about the blood (that there may be some, but it is not "hurt" blood); labor is hard work and faces sometimes look strange when they are working hard; noises, we also make some strange sounds when we work hard (grunts, etc.), and, also, the need for quiet and understanding. The children should see as many films, still pictures, and slides, as possible. Be sure to discuss where the baby comes from **exactly,** what it **is,** "the vagina" a special place for the baby to come out and that it is **not,** the place we urinate from or have a B.M. Explain the placenta and do it several times. Leave plenty of openings and invitations for questions. Have someone there responsible for the children (see paragraph 2 below). If your children are old enough to communicate and relate to other children, it is nice if they can talk to other children who have experienced the birth of a sibling.

2. **Child Caretakers.** You will be busy in labor and so will your husband. If children are to be present, there should be someone there to help them. They should know the children or have a chance, at least, to get to know them. They can also be your cameraman or have other functions, but should understand the children are the priority. They should know the children's routine, where their clothes are, special toys, food needs, anything that they enjoy doing, and be willing and able to help them and keep them company through labor and birth. Of corse, they should be prepared as any other adult present by attending **your** get-together, having **at least** seen birth films and having the love, empathy and understanding for **your** birth choice.

3. **Cameramen.** It is easier (from experience) to handle one camera. So if you want a film and stills, you would be better off with two people. (However it is **possible** for one person to do it.) They should know how you want your film shot (perineal view, side view, and so on), what story you want to impart, where you want your emphasis (on the mother's reaction, the coach's role, the children, the family that births together, and so on), anything you especially want left out (the perineum - you can get the birth and not the perineum), the placenta (some find it "yuckie"), and what you especially want in your film (your children's reaction to birth, yours, your husband's, the coaching, labor, the people who were at your birth). You will buy your film ahead of time. If you buy only a little, you should plan carefully how you want it used (for four total rolls, use one for labor, two for birth, and one for the party). In other words, don't leave it to them completely unless you really don't have any preferences. You can't go back and retake and you don't want to feel afterwards "Gee I wish I had pictures of . . . ." If you are not sure you want pictures, we love ours and can relive that magic moment many times over. Much of the birth (children's reaction, and so on) would have been missed without our precious photos. Again, cameramen must have the same preparation as already mentioned. You should have them at the meeting(s), a list, and a signal for them if you want them to stop filming at anytime. You should not feel bound if you are uncomfortable at anytime and don't wish the filming. This should be discussed beforehand.

4. **Birth Facilitator.** This person would be in charge of running errands for your coach (so he doesn't have to leave you), getting cool rags, ice chips, blankets, and so on, making any necessary meals, answering the phone or door, keeping people out when you want privacy, bringing them in when the birth is imminent, having emergency numbers and **your** plans in case of emergency, knowing how you want particulars planned in case of emergency (where children go, what if Mom has to go to emergency room what to do with baby, and so on), setting up the birthday party,

helping clean bedding afterwards, and checking the time at birth. As you can see, it would be much better if this person had some experience having been at births.

Do not misunderstand. All these jobs can be taken by one person, but that person should have prior experience as a birth facilitator or disaster could ensue. Two people are ideal as they can back each other. Too many, as mentioned before, can resemble a circus more than an intimate birth experience. If you have more people, they're just observing. Your birth facilitator should have enough authority to keep everyone out if this is your immediate desire. This should be done with no more than a hand signal, should be discussed and understood by all, and you should feel free enough with everyone there to exercise this right at any time.

A PROFESSIONAL SPEAKS

Children's Preparation for Birth

By CHERYL WINES, AAHCC

Having been a childbirth instructor for more than eight years for A.A.H.C.C., I strongly feel that parents, and anyone who is to attend a birth, be carefully prepared. In our society, birth is not a commonplace social happening. Most adults have never been exposed to anything but negatives related to birth. Although children's minds are less spoiled with negative attitudes, they still haven't the exposure that children in other cultures do.

In the capacity of friend and photographer, I have attended over 50 births, most of which had one or more siblings present. I have seen children ranging in ages from 18 months to 21 years sharing the birth of a sibling. I have seen one other sibling and as many as eight other siblings present at a birth. I have only once seen what I feel was not a positive experience for a sibling. That is probably why I have such definite feelings about "child preparation". This child was raised in a conservative home and was three-and-a-half years old. His parents had done **no** preparation at all. There was no one there specifically to take care of him. Everyone else had a specific job. When the baby was born, he was frightened at the blood and put off by the meconium the baby passed after birth. Seeing this, I tried to reassue him and was partially successful. His father finally picked him up and he was fine. Ever since that experience, many years ago, I have welcomed siblings to my film night in class and carefully outlined a suggested program for preparing siblings for birth.

Basically, this includes:

(1) Frequent discussion and verbal explanation of what to expect. Blood, water breaking (sometimes with a pop and splash), meconium, the placenta, vernix, and so on, should be carefully explained.

(2) Practicing in front of children frequently: Explaining contractions, Mom's need for quiet (and having the child practice **their** "role"). Mom can't talk, Dad's busy, and so on. Be realistic practicing

second stage — grunt! Make your face look like you're working. Remember your techniques may not be perfect. Children should be prepared for noises. Be sure and talk about the baby and the need for the child to be quiet so as not to scare the baby.

(3) A picture is worth a thousand words. Show as many pictures in as many mediums as possible. Films, stills, slides, etc. Point out in each, blood, placenta, meconium, vernix, and so on. All the things you've discussed.

(4) Especially for children under five years a caretaker specifically and exclusively for the child(ren) should be there. Don't assume you won't need help. Even my seven- and nine-year-olds at our last birth got bored waiting around midnight and decided to have a water balloon fight in the street. I never knew until well after the birth. (Then it was amusing!) Be sure the caretaker understands what you want. I've found at the birth it is best to allow the child to be wherever they want. It's much better because sometimes children (especially older children) will stand back. Younger children often want to be right in the action. Discuss how you feel about this and clear it with your birth attendant. Other than that, the caretaker should stand back and be ready to whisper any reassurances or answer questions for the child and watch carefully for concerned looks, and so on.

(5) Miscellaneous considerations:

A thought should be made to the child's acceptance of his mother's nudity. Don't mince words about exactly where the baby comes from.

After the birth you are engrossed in the baby, but your birth attendant may take the time to show older children the placenta and cord and how they work.

Try to accept your child's attitude, whatever it is. Remember a nonchalant reaction is usually a total natural acceptance of the whole process. Once the baby comes the child may be more interested in calling Grandma or eating the birthday cake. Be sure and include them without forcing them. Allow them to adjust and become acquainted in their own time.

From personal experience and observation there is no greater joy than sharing the birth of a baby with the perfect, natural, unaffected awe of a child. If you want to truly see nature, there is no better teacher of the appreciation of its beauty and simplicity than a child.

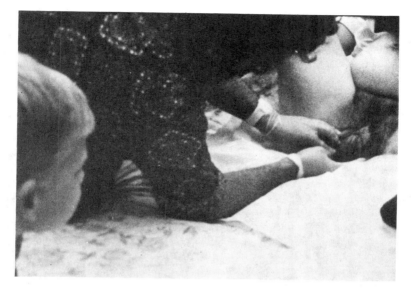

Aaron watches Wendy give birth.

KATHRYN GORMAN

Hello Kathryn

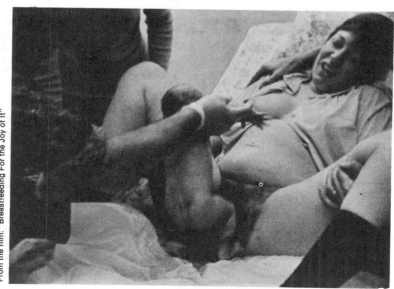

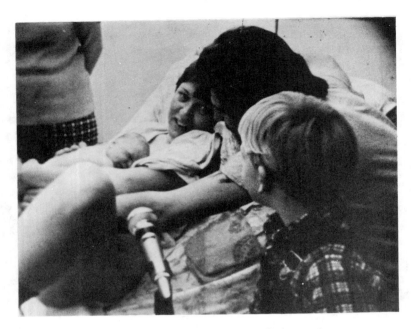

"I want her clean and dry, then I'll touch her"

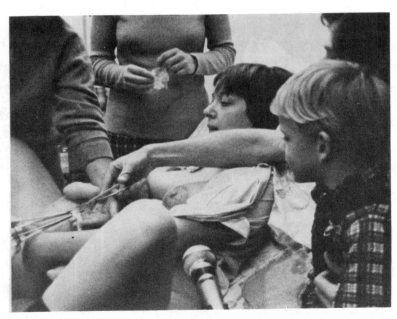

Cutting the Cord

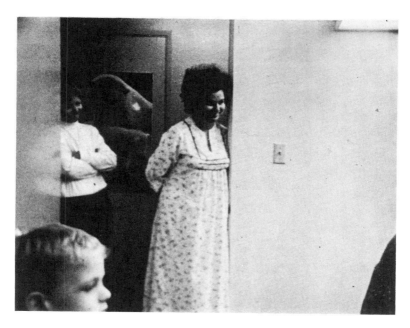

Grandma Came To Help

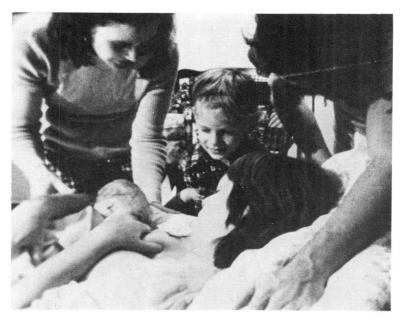

Nursing

The Actual Birth — How To Handle It

Preparing for the actual birth takes a lot of time, and a lot of thought. When will the birth occur? Where will it occur? How do you handle false alarms? What to do when the "real thing" starts? When do you tell the children? How to get them out of school? What stories will your children tell other children? Preparing for a home birth. Preparing for a hospital birth. When will the baby be born? Labor and Birth.

When will the birth occur? Day or night? You need to consider the regular patterns of your children. If you have a birth at night when your children normally sleep, you might want to wait until the last minute to awaken them. Of course, this depends on their ages. If they are very young, sleep may be the best thing. If they are old enough to help they may want you to wake them up and let them join in the preparations. During the day toddlers might like to play, rest, take a walk or nap (all under supervision.) Of course, older children might want to go to school, or stay home, depending on how sure you are about being in labor in the morning.

Sleep. This is important for everyone attending the birth. Sleepy people can be very fussy, and get on each other's nerves very quickly. For pregnant women, sleep can be essential. If you have not had enough sleep everything is exaggerated. The contractions seem harder and longer. Things that would not bother you, seem like major problems if you do not have enough sleep.

Pain is intensified if you do not have enough sleep, and you may not have enough energy to take care of your own baby after the birth. You may not be able to give birth but instead have to be delivered by forceps or cesarean section if you do not have enough sleep ahead of time. The last three months of pregnancy take a nap every day, if you can, and be sure you are rested at all times. If you think you are in early labor go to sleep. I have never heard of anyone sleeping through the actual birth.

False Alarms. Many women have what is called false labor or Braxton-Hicks labor. These are periods of contractions that may last for several hours and then stop. Generally speaking, if you change activity or do some pelvic rocks the contractions stop. Think of these times as practice for the real thing. These early contractions also help your baby by massaging it and preparing it for the outside world.

119

Real Labor. Having had six children, I will share with you what little I know about real labor. Keep in mind that labor usually does not start when you think it will. Here are some of the signs of labor:

1. **Nesting.** This is the time when you get a burst of energy and clean everything. This may go on for weeks or you may get an urge to clean everything just before the birth.

2. **Contractions.** Everyone gets these. They feel like a balloon blowing up inside of your abdomen or your abdomen gets hard all over. Your coaches should time contractions from the beginning of one to the beginning of the next. They also should time how long each contraction itself lasts. Perhaps even more important is that the contractions should get stronger in intensity. You may feel contractions in your abdomen, down low like menstrual cramps or in your lower back. In any case, someone putting their hand on your abdomen will feel it get hard and move forward during a contraction.

3. **Bloody Show.** When the cervix starts opening there is a mucus plug that comes out. If some of the small capillaries break at this time, there will be a bloody show. A bloody show all by itself does not mean anything. You may have a bloody show after an internal exam or after intercourse. If you have contractions and a bloody show that is a plus.

4. **Apparent Diarrhea.** Your body generally cleans itself out just before or in early labor.

5. **Malor Flush.** This is a flush that covers the cheek bones as labor starts to get down to business. It is most noticeable around four centimeters and gradually fades.

6. **Loss of Appetite.** As labor progresses you have less desire for food. If you have a long labor you may get hungry occasionally. Some birth centers now allow popsicles, tea, broth, 7-UP, and so on. Others allow you to eat a soft diet and some still say "nothing by mouth".

7. **Effacement.** This is when the cervix thins out. Your birth attendant judges this during an internal exam. How much thinning is gauged by percent.

8. **Dilation.** This is how far open the cervix is. Again this is determined during an internal exam. Dilation is measured in centimeters: 0 to approximately 10.

9. **The bag of waters breaking.** This can be a sign that labor is about to start in which case, call your doctor. In most cases the bag of waters does not break until second stage.

10. **Loss of Modesty.** This is another sign of labor. In the beginning the mother has the covers up to her chin. As labor progresses the covers get lower and lower until she no longer cares if she is covered at all. At this point the birth is not far away.

11. **Inability to talk during contractions.**

12. **Intuition.** This is perhaps one of the best indicators and no one can say why.

When will labor begin? No one really knows but these signs may help you.

Home birth preparation should be done well in advance. Go over the supplies you will need with your birth attendant. One thing the children can help with is making the birth bed. First make your bed as you usually would, then place some kind of waterproof cover on top of this and make the bed again. This way you have clean sheets already made up for after the birth. They are protected and can be snuggled into. Three different types of waterproof protection are: 1. Plastic painting drop cloths, generally available at paint stores for less than a dollar; 2. Plastic material like the kind used for table cloths; or 3. Flannel covered rubberized sheeting— this comes cut into crib sizes or by the yard.

Hospital births. This takes just as much thought. Take a tour of the hospital you are going to. Learn about all the procedures they consider routine. Explain them to the children so that they are not frightened by them. Meet the personnel. This makes everyone more at ease when the time comes to enter the hospital. Take along quiet play things: toys, books, games, etc. If the hospital allows, take

No matter where you have your baby you need to let everyone know what your wishes are. We did this by writing a letter that our children passed out to everyone who came . . .

Dear Special Friends,

Welcome to our special Birth-Day Party. We are very happy you could help us celebrate the birth of a very special person. We invite you to join us in the festivities after the birth and have a good time.

Since we cannot predict when you will arrive or when our special surprise guest will arive, or what condition of work Jay or Marjie will be in, we have taken the liberty of writing down some of the ground rules and some of our thoughts about this birth.

The interim name for the baby at this time is Elsie. This will not be the name after the birth but we feel better being able to call the baby by name . We choose Elsie because she or he kicked like a cow.

Last year at this time we had a miscarriage after 5 months of pregnancy, so it seems like we have been pregnant for 17 months this time around. The children say it is not fair for a mother to have two 1st trimesters.

The baby this time is weeks late, which has had its effect on everyone's nerves. At least we hope the birth occurs during a time when all the family will be able to be present.

It is very important to us that our children be involved in this birth. We ask that they have the "Front Row Seats". We also ask that no one touch or wipe the baby off until Jay and the children have had their chance.

We may want periods of total privacy. This may mean you may be asked to step out for awhile. TV - Video Tape, Computer games and such are available for your enjoyment. Help yourself to food and drink.

We are very pleased that Vic and Salee Berman will be on hand if needed for Medical help, but we hope that Medical Intervention will not be necessary and that Medical Supplies and equipment will be kept out of sight (if near-by)

Some of our wishes may seem different to you. Because we want no exams, none of us may know exactly what is happening at some times, however, you realize that even WITH exams...you still never know for sure. Also, we want a cool room to birth in, films and movies, no gloves, and I am sure other things that may sound strange to you. I am sure if Jay is not busy he will be happy to explain our reasons.

We feel strongly that "It's not nice to fool mother nature" and we want to follow our feelings and have as natural birth as possible.

Thank you for sharing this with us.

Love,

Jay, Marjie, Odell, Susan. Coni, JJ, Bobby, and Elsie

a portable TV especially if they have a lounge where the children can play. Bring food the children like from home. Keep a cooler in the car for munchies. Be sure there is a place where the children can sleep — a lounge or car — if it is during their regular sleep or nap time. Also check out places the children can play or run, under the supervision of your babysitter. Is there a park nearby or is the parking lot generally empty? Children should never be left alone or unsupervised. If they are kept inside without exercise for a long labor they may get very uncontrollable. Check out the facilities for camera equipment.

Pain is frequently a part of birth. How big a part depends on preparation ahead of time. Let's look at some of the causes of pain.

1. Fear especially of the unknown. Sometimes this can also be fear of a past experience or past birth. Fear causes adrenalin to be produced by the body and the contractions may stop or become ineffective.
2. Tension causes pain by fighting or tensing up against what nature is trying to do. Total relaxation is the answer to tension.
3. Chest breathing can cause tension and a feeling of panic or fear. Chest breathing robs a woman of the energy she needs in labor.
4. Fatigue causes anything to be exaggerated. Contractions feel worse. Things bother you more. Get lots of sleep toward the end of pregnancy.
5. Disobeying the laws of nature. Read the chapter in "Husband-Coached Childbirth" on "It's not nice to fool Mother Nature". Anytime you interfere with the natural process there are consequences.
6. Something wrong. Pain is the body's way of telling you something is wrong. If the pain is overwhelming, perhaps the labor should be re-evaluated for the cause.
7. Interference in any way with a laboring woman can cause pain. Even a conversation can distract her and cause pain, let alone vaginal exams and physical interferences.
8. Chemical intervention can cause pain. Inductions and stimulations of labor with drugs often cause more pain than normal births.
9. The birth itself is sometimes painful but generally controllable if there is proper support and coaching.

Ways to handle pain:

1. **Relaxation.** These are techniques you should practice every day. We have given you some in this book and I am sure you will learn more.
2. **Dissociation.** Use the word contraction instead of pain.
3. **Cognitive rehearsal.** This means rehearse everything that will go on — what will happen in labor; what will the coach do; and what will the children do. Try to cover all the bases.
4. **Hawthorne Effect.** This is the effect of personal attention. For this reason it is important to get into small classes and it is

important to have lots of personal attention at the birth. Everyone does a better job if they have personal attention.

5. Medication is another way to handle pain, but from the mothers I have talked to, it is generally not very effective. This has also been my experience. One couple who had been given a drug during labor had very different ideas on its effectiveness. The husband believed that the drug was very useful and helped his wife a lot. She stopped complaining and was quiet. When the wife got to talk she said the medication did **nothing** for the pain but simply made her quiet!

Bonding should be a family experience. Before you can understand bonding there are certain things one must observe. First of all, newborn babies can see, they can follow, they can locus. I know there are many textbooks that tell you they cannot but these authors either have never observed a natural childbirth baby, or have observed babies after they have had silver nitrate put into their eyes. If silver nitrate is used, it can be delayed! In California the law says it must be put into the eyes in the first two hours. I suggest waiting that two hours. It gives the baby a chance to see Mommie, Daddy and its brothers and sisters.

Seeing and looking each other in the eye, so to speak, is very important. You know when someone looks at you and you know when you have made contact with another person by eye-to-eye contact. New babies bond in this way to their family.

Touch is another way of bonding. Right after birth there is a moment or two of surprise or disbelief. Everyone has to realize that this is really a baby and it is really alive. Then I notice that the mother and father are generally the first to touch the baby. Brothers and sisters generally start out slowly by touching first the fingers or toes working their way cautiously to the body of the baby. Children need to understand why the baby is wet, hot, and has (may have) a white cheesey substance on it and why it may be bloody. Some children may prefer to wait until the baby is cleaned up before touching it. This is fine.

Smell is another way of bonding for the newborn. The baby can smell and very quickly knows the smell of its mother. The baby can tell the difference between another baby's mother and its own just by smell. In one study gauze that was in the mother's bra was placed in front of the newborn baby's nose. The baby started sucking movements when the gauze placed in front of it was from its own mother but not from another mother's. I am sure babies know the smell of their siblings. I know Ann will stay asleep when handed from family member to family member but will awaken if handed to someone outside of the family.

Feel is another way of bonding. The newborn is very sensitive to this and responds to the feel of skin, blankets, water and such. At many births I have attended, the parents and children take off their shirts just to be able to bond to the new baby by skin-to-skin contact.

Sound is a way of bonding also. The newborn baby has had a lot of experience hearing, long before it is born. The baby hears inside the uterus. In reading about experiments with sound underwater we know that sound travels better in water than it does in air. The baby is used to its mother's voice and internal noises. In Japan they recorded the noises inside the uterus and played this back to newborn babies. The recording soothed babies in the nursery but the recording had to be played very loud for this effect to happen. So loud that the Nursery room nurses found it uncomfortable for **them**. So the mother's voice is very important to the baby. Putting the baby on the mother's breast also allows the baby to hear the heartbeat of the mother. Other voices may also be important since babies do react inside the uterus to loud noises.

Breastfeeding also bonds the baby. The sucking is very important to the baby for nourishment, development, and comfort.

Breastfeeding is so much a part of natural childbirth that I feel it is also important to the family. Breastfeeding is so easy and natural. If you want some good basic information on breastfeeding go to La Leche Meetings and read their book "The Womanly Art of Breastfeeding." I also suggest you see the film "Breastfeeding for the JOY of It." This film goes into some of the basics of breastfeeding.

Be sure you have the proper position for nursing. Put the baby's head in the crook of your arm with your hand and arm down the back and buttocks. Be sure the nipple gets into the baby's mouth as far as possible. If you are engorged, express a few drops of milk to get the nipple elongated and easier to put into the baby's mouth. If for some reason you have to take the baby off the breast, be sure you break the suction first by placing your finger between the corner of the baby's mouth and the breast.

Remember your milk supply is a matter of supply and demand. The more often you nurse, the more milk you will have. If your baby is wetting six to eight diapers a day it is probably getting plenty of milk. Babies do have growth spurts and your baby may want to nurse more often at times. Newborn babies frequently nurse every 20 minutes! This generally lengthens out until the baby has a growth spurt and wants to nurse frequently again for a few days. Most babies have rest periods during a 24-hour period. These periods may be several hours. Take advantage of them and sleep yourself. Breastfeeding can be a family time. Young brothers and sisters may really enjoy it if you read to them at this time or they might like to read to you.

HAWAIIAN FAMILY BIRTHING

Our interest in the natural process, and our love of Hawaii has led us to investigate the birth practices of the Hawaiians — a culture untouched by the European modes of medicine until 200 years ago.

"When I was 9 years old, I helped my aunt at a birth. I enthusiastically told a white neighbor that Mrs. D. had 'borned a new baby', and the following day my mother was visited by a delegation of four white women who told her it was not 'nice' for me to know of such things."

On the day of birth (hanau) many relatives gathered. The expectant mother was urged to walk to and fro in labor. A reddish-colored amniotic fluid meant a boy, brownish meant a girl, thick fluid meant a large baby. A baby that took too

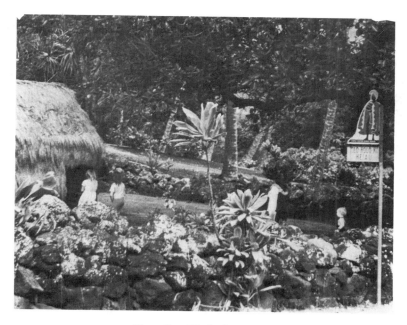

Hawaiian Birth Center

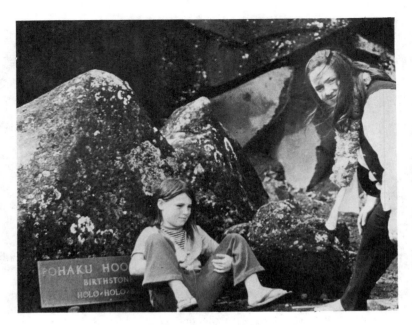

Hawaiian Delivery Room

long was said to be "kalilolilo" (snatching at life). The tree under which the placenta was buried became the property of the child.

The first movements were always noted. If the child turned to face the mother, the child would always love her. The grandparent cleaned the babies mouth with a finger. The grandparent "in charge" sucked the nose of the baby, after rinsing his mouth. There was NO substitute for mother's milk.

So, you see, the family all helped ... from the grandparents to the kids. Perhaps we could learn a thing ot two from the Hawaiians.

Freely adapted from:
   "Hawaiian Beliefs and Customs During Birth"
   by Mary Kawena Pukui
   From Bishop Museum Occasional Papers
   March 20, 1942

GRANDPARENTS
AT BIRTH

At a recent conference Dr. Mayer Eisenstein asked the audience "How many of you would want your mother at your birth?" and a few people raised their hands. Then he asked "How many would like to be their when your daughter has a baby" and almost every hand went up.

This is the generation gap ... think about it. What a tragedy! It is possible that bonding can be extended to the whole family? To multiple generations? Isn't this what life is all about?

At NAPSAC Dr. Eisenstein said, "We have to start this family bonding right now. We have to start strengthening the family. We have been doing this for over a year and a half. The majority of women have had either their mother or mother-in-law with them. The have always greatly supported the laboring woman, greatly supported their son or son-in-law, and always made the birth experience one of elation ... we have to learn not to split families. We have to learn not to be independent. We have to learn to be dependent. LIFE IS SO HARD, and we should try to seek as many people as we can to help us."

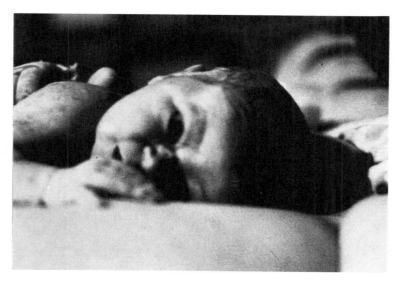

TOM GREENING, Ph.D.

Interview with Tom Greening, Ph.D., Psychologist, Father of two.

T. It is important to stress that the child be intellectually and emotionally prepared for what's going to happen, just as we prepare the expectant mother and father. They have somne sense of the sequence; who's doing what and why. Then if something unexpected, painful, medically difficult or bloody happens, there must be a way in which the child can, quickly as possible, deal with it, by asking questions of some adult, getting information, being held and reassured. Of course, at all times the child must have permission to leave and must have an environment where he still can be safe.

For a young child especially there should be a baby sitter available. I believe the basic principle would be to give the child control or mastery of the experience through intellectual and emotional preparation, through freedom of choice about staying or leaving, through having access to supportive adults. The biggest negative thing to avoid would be for the child to have a sense of helplessness in the face of powerful and mysterious events.

I think children have great resources to enjoy and understand events and to tolerate even stressful events as long as they do not feel overwhelmed or trapped.

M. That's very good.

T. Another obvious point would be to know the pre-existing health and status of the child's relationship to the mother and father, and to anyone else present. If the mother has a painful and difficult birth and if a child has experienced a lot of friction with his mother, he may feel guilty for being a bad child and hurting the mother. This could get a child pretty upset.

A child who may have had a tenuous bond to a mother might feel endangered of losing her. Here again, the need for support and including the child as much as possible, interacting with the child and giving the child an active participating role whenever possible, is important. The fact must also be faced that toward the final stages of birth, the child may be on his own and not get support from the mother and father for a short period.

M. That's where the adult comes in.

T. As for the preparation, I wouldn't want this to be the first time the child ever saw his mother undressed. Being part of the pregnancy and being prepared is important to prevent jealousy. We would want to try to anticipate and prevent any feelings of jealousy and abandonment.

M. Children feel part of it if they're there.

T. Yes, I believe the psycho-analytic nonsense about the trauma of witnessing the birth or witnessing the parents having intercourse has been overstated. It depends upon the pre-existing relationship between the child and parent, the way in which the child interrupts the event, and the way in which the event is interpreted to the child.

     M. Do you think that it would cause damaging sexual problems for a teenager possibly?

T. If the teenager were at that very moment guiltily obsessed or confused about sex, it could be a problem. Hopefully, with good communication, the parents would be aware of that. Some children might feel "I don't know who I am," "I am overwhelmed with the whole idea of sexuality and a woman's body," "I don't want any more; I can't handle that," or "I want to go play baseball."

     M. The choice, then, should be made by the child.

T. I believe kids tend to know what choices feel good to them.

VICTOR BERMAN, M.D.
SALEE BERMAN, R.N.

Interview with Victor Berman, M.D. and Salee Berman, R.N., Founders of NACHIS, Natural Childbirth Institute, Culver City, California, Parents of six.

M. How do you feel about children being present at births? Do you allow it in your birth center?

V. Yes, we definitely allow children. We've had 329 births in the birth center.

J. Does that count us?

S. Yes.

V. Of the 329 births about two-thirds were having their first baby, and one-third were multips. That's the original breakdown. It's changing now towards more multips. Of the one-third that are multips, at least half of them have had other children with them.

J. About one-sixth of the whole group?

V. That makes a sixth of the whole group, or over 50. We've had them have very young children — one-and-a-half years, two years — and we have had them as old as 16 and 17 years of age.

M. Have you had any problems with them?

V. Not a single problem. The only problem is in taking care of young children. Somebody has to take care of them because they run wild; their parents are naturally preoccupied.

S. We have set up certain criteria which we feel would be better if parents would follow when considering bringing siblings, or other children to the birth. Number one, the children should go to childbirth classes with them. They should see as many films and pictures of birth scenes and understand what the parents are doing. Their parents should talk openly about what's going to happen at the birth. We really like them to bring the children down to the open house so they can actually see a film of a birth. We actually want them to have an adult there at the center with the child, someone who the child can relate to — somebody who can read to him, or play with him, or take care of him when he's bored and reassure him that everything is going well. Because his parents are involved in the birth, they need to know that their other children are not being frightened and that their needs are being cared for.

V. Most people are concerned about what's going to frighten children, what's going to leave a wrong impression. They try to protect children from everything that goes on. I believe that if everyone would just remember his own childhood — the things they've heard, saw and thought which were never explained. Many of

131

these childhood impressions last throughout your life. People have talked about being frightened of things which seem silly when they look back at them as an adult; being frightened of childbirth, specifically. It's as simple as hearing somebody talk about someone bleeding or someone almost dying. I've heard several times that my mother almost died when I was born. They would tell me, when I was young, that my mother had a semi or half a cesarean. I never questioned it until I got older. What is half a cesarean? There is, of course, no such thing. But I believed this until I was in high school, or college, or medical school. I don't remember exactly.

This is the kind of misinformation children pick up. They are not going to pick up misinformation like that if they are invited participants to a birth and they are aware of what's happening. They can ask questions about it; they will ask questions about it.

S. Today this three-and-a-half-year-old was looking around. Then he asked, "Why is he wearing a rubber glove?"

V. That was the only question he had.

    M. Vic, as an obstetrician who has assisted a number of births with children present, what is your role? Do you explain to them what's happening if they're interested?

V. Yes. Children are very interested in what's taking place — why the baby looks crinkly — why the baby looks blue — why the baby sneezes — why the baby coughs — why the baby's wet — what's the placenta — what's the umbilical cord? Depending on their age, they will accept all of this on varying levels, from a very simple level for the very young to a good scientific explanation for the older kids.

I must emphasize again that I have never seen any sign whatsoever of any child being afraid, abnormally disturbed or hysterical. Frequently, they see blood — they want to know why there's blood. They see pain — they want to know why there's pain. I always encourage the mother to explain to them between contractions that it hurts, that it's painful; but reassure them that everything is all right and that it is worth the pain they feel. Certainly if they see the beautiful result afterward, the pain doesn't bother them. Kids are attuned to pain. They are always falling down, getting cut, scrapping their chins, knees and elbows, and getting bloody noses. This is part of being a child. A little bit of blood doesn't bother a child, nor does a little bit of pain.

    M. Do you think that this could possibly cause any sexual problems with teenagers?

V. I really don't think so. It's simply part of the relationships that different couples have with their children in different ways. I'm not advising anyone to bring their children. For those children who are ready and for those parents that want to bring them, I can't imagine any trouble. I do not recommend that a child be forced to witness a birth if they do not want to.

    M. Salee, as the mother of teenagers, have your children ever been at a birth?

S. Of course.

    M. Have you encountered any problems because of it?

S. No. All of our children have seen births. Their ages range from 31 to 12 and, of course, they have seen births when they were much younger. The fact is that the two younger children are very interested in birth. They both want to be doctors.

ERIC GUTNICK, M.D.

Interview with Eric Gutnick, M.D., Obstetrician, Fort Bragg, California. Mendocino Coast Hospital is 160 miles north of San Francisco. Since 1975 they have encouraged children at births.

M. Tell me how did you get started doing this?

E. Basically we cover a large area of the Northern California coast. There are about 20 deliveries here a month in the hospital, and a number of other deliveries in the community at home which we do not attend. We do prenatal care for people who want home births. We have lay midwives in the area. Also, in our office we have three obstetricians and one certified nurse-midwife. We do hospital births. The way deliveries are set up it's not an alternative birth center. Everyone's basically handled the same way. The labor happens in one of the regular hospital rooms with windows and regular beds. The birth happens in this bed. Usually we have a bean bag chair and a little nice comfortable pillow for the woman to sit on. Reasonable sterile techniques are used in terms of gowns and gloves. The father can participate in the delivery and, usually after the head is out, he can deliver the rest of the baby if he wishes. The mother gets to hold the baby immediately after birth and can also breastfeed the baby at that time.

That's assuming everything is normal. If there are any abnormalities, we can do fetal monitoring and whatever else is appropriate. Everyone has taken childbirth classes. It is extremely unusual to need any medication during labor. Sometimes if an episiotomy is needed, we use a local. Otherwise, its unusual to require anything at all. People can decide what they want in terms of delivery, whether they want the baby to have a bath, and so on. Their friends and children can be there if they wish.

M. How did you get into the children being there?

E. It just seemed like a natural thing. Past births had happened at home and the rest of the family was there. It's a family experience. During the prenatal visits, we encourage pregnant women to bring their partners. They can also bring their children to learn what's happening, where the baby's at, and where it comes out, and what babies look like when they are born. It seems like a good bond to establish. We like another adult to be there to supervise the children in case there are any problems. We like them to have some instruction so they know where babies come from, to see a film on childbirth before, and go over what will happen in labor. Explain to the child that although the mother seems uncomfortable, it is just part of the natural process, as is the bleeding. Babies do not come out dressed up and shining. If they are not aware of all this, seeing the blood can freak out little children who are unaware of what's happening. If a Cesarean section is required, the father can be in the operating room. However, the children are not permitted there.

M. Do the children and father gown up?

E. The children do not have gowns. They must wash their hands before the birth. The father, however, has to gown up if he is going to take part in the birth.

M. How do you get around the health department?

E. We have sought their approval. That's the reasonable way to do it. The mother stays in the same room in which she delivers. She's not moved anywhere. Most of the women stay either overnight or go home the same day after about eight hours. There has been no increase in infection in terms of either normal deliveries or C-sections with the father present. It has worked out very well.

M. You have found no increase of infections as far as the children are concerned?

E. No, we haven't.

M. Do you screen the children for colds, chicken pox, and so forth?

E. Yes. They are screened for that.

M. I assume that most mothers are breastfeeding?

E. Almost all. It is very important.

M. Do you feel that other hospitals could do this same thing?

E. Other hospitals that wanted to could probably do it. I think many of them don't want to.

M. They tell me it's against the law?

E. I think that is because no one tries to change it. We have gotten permission to do it and it has worked out well.

M. Have you had any bad experiences with children being there?

E. I wouldn't say any bad experiences at all. Most of them have been very postive.

M. Many people feel that viewing their mother in this condition will cause sexual problems with children later on. How do you feel about this?

E. In this community it is very common for a woman to bring in both small and large children with them when they come in for their regular pelvic examinations, birth control pills, and prenatal visits. They are well aware of what's happening and know where everything goes. I can't image that it can cause more problems than there are sexual problems already in the country.

KITTIE FRANTZ, R.N.

Interview with Kittie Frantz, R.N. Pediatric Nurse Practitioner, La Lache League Leader, Mother of Three

M. Jay said you had attended a birth and maybe you could tell us about it.

K. I was working at the NACHIS Birth Center. The mother had been in labor for a while and there was a eight-to-ten-year-old child there who had come along for the birth. I was busy seeing patients. Some of my patients didn't show up so I had some free time. I was talking with the Dad and he was explaining how he prepared the child. They had talked about it and he had gone with them to the Bradley classes. We were all talking excitedly about how the baby was coming and how she wanted it to be a boy. The midwife came out and said, "It's getting close." Everyone scurried back into the birth room.

The father made a mad dash into the room and the child disintegrated into tears and retreated back into the waiting room which was empty. I went and sat down next to her, put my arm around her and asked her what was wrong. She said that she was afraid and she really didn't want to see the birth. I was having difficulty finding out exactly what she was afraid of. I was assuming that, at her age, she did not want to see her mother in pain.

Someone came out and said, "You better hurry if you want to see the baby born." She started to go and then pulled back. I said, "Would you like me to go with you and we'll stand at the door." She seemed receptive to that. We walked to the door of the birth room. Then I knelt to her height and explained that "your Mommy is working hard." At one point I looked up at the mother whose face was contorted because she was pushing hard. I realized that it was having an effect on the child. I said, "Smile, Mom, or people might think you're in pain." The mother quickly picked up on the cue. People started explaining what the mother was doing. They said things like, "Isn't Mommy pushing hard." The child began to relax a little bit and pick up on the excitment of the birth. She saw the actual birth and everything went quite well.

Afterwards the mother thanked me for taking the time to help her child through that. The mother said she felt helpless because she was so tied up with the birth and she knew that her other child had a need that she couldn't fulfill. One of the birth attendants said, "That's exactly why we have a rule here that a child that attends a birth must attend with a person that the child really enjoys." We can't have unattended children at birth. Another adult or an older sibling, someone that can guide the child through the experience, should be there. If the child were having second thoughts, or if there was a toddler at the birth, they could make sure that they weren't in the other room pulling the syringes out of the drawers.

M.   Have you had a chance to talk to the mother since?

K.   Yes, I followed the baby pediatrically for a little while. The little girl came in. There seemed to be a really strong bond between the little girl and myself.

PAUL FLEISS, M.D.

Interview with Paul Fleiss, M.D., F.A.A.P., Pediatrician, Father of six.

M. Dr. Fleiss what do you think of having children present at birth?

P. The baby is part of the family. Unless there's a medical problem, I think it's important to have the whole family there. I don't see any danger except in case of medical emergencies. Children need to be prepared for the small chance of some kind of catastrophy or a deformed baby.

M. When you and Elissa had your most recent baby did you have your children present?

P. Of course. All five of our children were present. Of course, they were not there all the time. The birth was about 1:30 in the morning and we woke the kids up as the baby was crowning. Then all five of our kids — they range in age from 8-14 came and welcomed him into the world. They were right there when he was born to hold and touch him, and they have a special place in their lives for him.

M. How important is preparation?

P. I think it's vital! I think if the mother isn't prepared and is not having natural childbirth, I would not want the children to watch the old fashioned childbirth, with blood and guts spilling out. Then I think they shouldn't be there.

M. Is there any risk to having children at birth?

P. I think if the kids are sick, coughing or sneezing they should wear a little mask or not be present. I don't think anyone who's sick should be at a birth. The kids can be instructed not to cough or sneeze on the baby, and they can understand why this is important. After all in a newborn baby a cold can be a disaster.

M. Some people fear children may be traumatized, have nightmares or future sexual problems if they witness a birth.

P. I think that's possible if they are unprepared. They need to understand about sex and childbirth, I was 12 or 13 before I knew about sex and birth. Childbirth education has to be for the whole family.

Breastfeeding is really important because it helps to pass on to the child special immunities that are present in the early milk or colostrum and in mother's milk through-out breastfeeding.

I think education is really important for us all. The more you learn about life and living, the better you are able to enjoy it. Children can learn about life and living by being present when life begins.

ODELL'S STORY

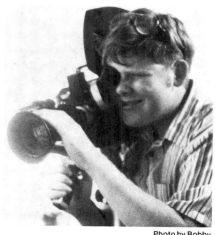

Odell "Me and my camera were ready"

It all started about eight years ago when my brother Bobby was born. I remember the morning my Mom went to the hospital. I remember the apprehension as we watched them drive off. I remember being alone in the house, wondering what was really happening, feeling the way a father must as he waits alone in a hospital waiting room. Then the telephone call from Dad telling us that Bobby was born. I remember that night when my Mom came home and told us that Bobby's birth was some sort of a miracle. They had thought that the baby was dead while she was in labor because they could not hear the fetal heart tones. I wondered then, what could I have done if I had been there? I also remember wanting to be there.

Then, there was the time Erving was aborted. My Mom had an extremely hard pregnancy. One day, without any warning, I came home to find my Mom and Dad not here. At first I wondered where they were. I remember that awful call from my Dad telling me that the baby had been aborted and my Mom was about to go into surgery. I remember the thoughts that ran through my mind, seeing the emotions on my brothers' and sisters' faces as I had to inform each and every one of them.

Next, December, on our way home from Asilomar, we learned quite accidentally that Mom was pregnant with Elsie. During that long and scarey pregnancy we wondered if Elsie would be a carbon copy of Erving.

One evening before leaving for Fremont High School to play in a band concert, we called home to make sure Mom wasn't in labor. Dad told us everything was perfectly okay. As Dad hung up the phone, my Mom said, "I think I'm in labor." Coming home later from the show, we learned Mom **was** in labor. At this news we began to prepare for the birth. We cleaned the house more thoroughly than usual, set up the camera equipment, put special sheets on the bed, and then settled back to wait. Around nine o'clock we had some disgusting pizza and finally everyone went to bed.

The next morning, I don't even know what time it was — the sun hadn't come up yet. I was the third person to be wakened. A number of people had been invited

139

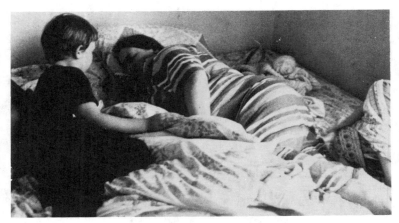

Bobby helps Mommy relax

to see this glorious event. I remember the people coming in and the joy in their faces and the sun slowly dawning on us. Of course, me and my camera were ready to film this event. While we waited, we watched some video tapes to pass the time.

At midday Susan, Bobby and I started working to help Mom, while Dad, Vic and Salee tried to figure out why the baby had not been born at five o'clock in the morning. Finally, around four that afternoon Vic broke the bag of waters. It was not just meconium stained, it was practically all meconium.

Then I had to go back to the front room and inform the guests that Vic was considering giving an IV. A little while later, I told the guests that Vic was now thinking about taking Mom either to a hospital or the birth center, and of course, making the arangements that I felt necessary for drivers and stuff. I had some drivers' training at the time, but I hadn't yet received my license.

The decision to go to the birth center which was close to the hospital came about an hour later. As we drove down to the center, my sisters were all crying on each other's shoulders. I watched my Mom's car intently from Salee's car as we drove.

At the birth center, we worked and coached my Mom. All of us were coaching. After about an hour, Ann was finally born. We later learned that the prolonged labor had been because her arm was stuck against her head, requiring the area in which she was born to be twice its normal size. That slowed down the birth process.

I remember feeling Ann, rubbing her. She was very warm and sticky. I remember my mother's face of pure joy even though she had spent the last several hours in tremendous pain. All the crying and suffering had now turned to joy at the sight of the newborn child.

As I look at Ann now, I see a healthy, alert baby — more alert than most children are at her age. Is it because Mom didn't have any drugs during her labor that she's like this? The answer came back to me — yes. I see no side effects in myself from this experience. I think the pure joy that we saw after the birth would convince anyone that it was worth it. Even my Mom says it's worth it. It was unfortunate that Ann's arm got stuck like that. Things like that happen just once-in-a-billion births. It was just a minor complication that took longer to deliver.

BOBBY HATHAWAY
An Interview (Age 8)

Bobby: Ann Elizabeth Minniedell Hathaway's birth was 35 hours.
Mother: Did you want to be there?
Bobby: Yes.
Mother: Do you think other children should be at their brother's and sister's births?
Bobby: Yes.
Mother: How old were you when Ann was born?
Bobby: Eight.
Mother: What did you think about when I was in labor?
Bobby: I thought you were in a lot of pain.
Mother: Did that bother you?
Bobby: No.

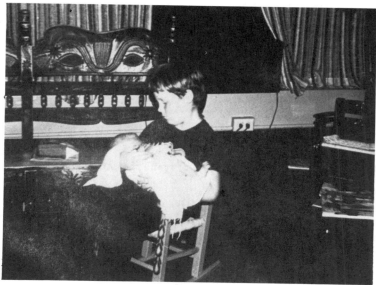

Photo by Connie

Bobby rocks Ann (her first rock)

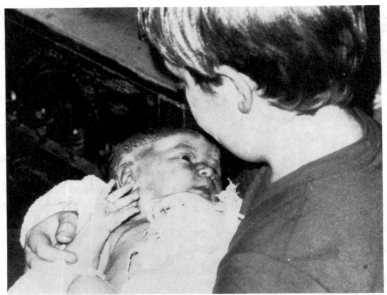

Bonding is for brothers, too

Mother:	What did you do during labor?
Bobby:	Sat around, took pictures.
Mother:	How were you prepared for this birth?
Bobby:	I saw movies, I went to a birth, we talked about it.
Mother	Why was Ann's birth so long?
Bobby:	Because her elbow was in the way.
Mother:	What did Ann look like when she was born?
Bobby:	All bloody.
Mother:	How soon did you touch her?
Bobby:	A couple of minutes after she was born.
Mother:	What did she feel like?
Bobby:	All yukkie and hot.
Mother:	Did you see the cord and placenta?
Bobby:	Hey, we should have a picture of the placenta in this story.
Mother:	How soon after birth did you rock Ann?
Bobby:	An hour-and-a-half.
Mother:	Do you like Ann?
Bobby:	Yep.
Daddy:	I think your story is all ready to print.
Bobby:	Yep, it's a good one.

SUSAN'S STORY

(Age 14)

As a child who has been present at three labors, present at two births and an active part of one birth, I think I've learned a lot about the feelings children might have towards birth.

One labor was at the birth center and it didn't work out; the mother had to be taken to the hospital. We (my father, 7-year-old brother and I) decided to go to the birth center after a phone call telling us the baby should be born by 6:00 p.m. (I have since learned babies can't tell time), and would we like to come? When we got there, nothing was going on. We had dinner and Bobby and I drew on the chalk board.

We decided that births were boring. Nobody had ever told me how boring it can be. In all the movies they just show the exciting parts - they don't tell you that it's 12 hours of "boring" for every one hour of excitment.

We finally fell asleep on the floor. About two in the morning we woke up to the lady's mother, who was upset, and was sure that her daughter and grandchild would surely die before completing a natural childbirth. This might have scared any other child but Bobby and I knew better than that. We knew that if anything was really wrong Dr. Berman would take her to the hospital and take care of the problem. Nothing could be that drastically wrong if she was still here. And nothing **was** that wrong, not at that point anyway. So we waited around another three hours while she was pushing. Dr. Berman decided to take her to the hospital as a precaution because she was not progressing as fast as usual. I felt sorry for the lady and her mother but I was just as happy to go home. But it upset Bobby more than I realized.

When the time came that we could go to the birth center to try again, Bobby refused to go. He said it was all his fault that the baby wouldn't come out. After about 15 minutes of reasuring him that it wasn't his fault he decided to try again. This birth worked out and was beautiful. The baby was born about 6:00 a.m. and we stood around watching for about a half an hour after the birth. (I would have cried but Dad had a camera in his hand.) We left because I had to be at school by 8:00 and it was a 45-minute drive from where we were. I went home and told Mom how great it was then I went to school and told EVERYONE. They all thought I was crazy!!

Then Mom got pregnant again. Seven years after Bobby. We had been teasing her for years about how she should have another baby. About a week before she told me she thought she was pregnant, we had given up and decided

143

that it was hopeless and we'd never get a new brother or sister. So when she told me I just about dropped my teeth!! Anyway that pregnancy ended up in a miscarriage which, at least for me, was very unexpected!! And I still cry when I think about it.

A few months later Mom got pregnant again and I feel that Ann and I are much closer than any sisters could ever be. I feel special because I heard her heartbeat first and I just used my ear. Nobody could hear it before that even with a stethoscope!

Ann's birth was very hard. After falling asleep on the bus coming home with the band from a football game and dreaming that Mom had the baby and then finding out she was in labor when we got home, I got nervous that we might have missed it. As you know it was a long hard labor and between brushing Mom's hair, getting her fruit juice and reassuring everyone else that everything was all right, I'd run outside and cry. I was very SCARED!

A lot of it had to do with the miscariage just months before. The reason I ran outside was because I was afraid everyone would laugh at me. I finally realized that the people that were here were the people that I trusted the most and felt closest to in the world. It helped when Lisa told me that it was all right.

When Mom let them break her bag of waters I was MAD because I thought she was just tired and would regret it later! Then she decided to go to the birth

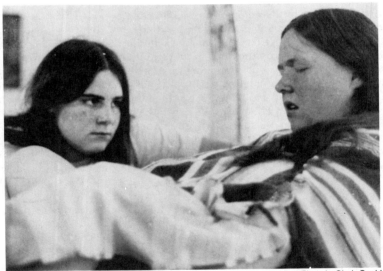

Photo by Gloria Goold

Susan supports Mommy

center. I got together everyone's phone number so that we could call them from the hospital to reveal the outcome. (At that point I was sure she would end up in the hospital.)

When we got to the birth center Dr. Berman said just one contraction then

144

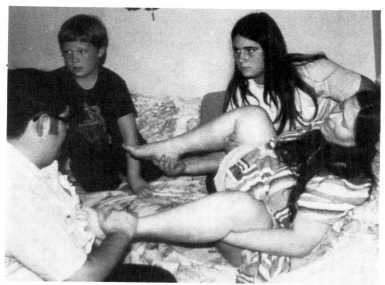

Photo by JJ

we'd go to the hospital. After about 10 contractions with Mom screaming that he lied and she really needed the hospital, he promised that she'd just have to go through a couple more then he'd take her to the hospital. And after five more contractions I was ready to hit him!

I kept thinking he'd be sorry if she died right there! At this point I was so scared I just held her hand, prayed and cried. And when she saw me crying she stopped screaming and said it was all right. (Now that threw me!) But I was still mad. How could these people let her go through this? I wished God would give me some of the pain so that she would have less.

Everyone kept saying that they could see the baby's head. Mom kept saying that they were lying. I thought they were too. When she finally came out I was in a state of shock. I couldn't believe it was a baby and it wasy alive. It moved. It cried and it was a GIRL! The first thing I remember about seeing Ann was when she looked up at Mom,the same way Mom had looked at me 15 minutes before saying everything was all right.

Ann is beautiful, Mom is beautiful and everything is all right. I've learned a lot about how some things just don't work out and some things are easy, but the best things you have to work for. And Ann is the best thing God has ever given us.

A few hours later when we finally got home Mom told us that she wanted someone to stay up with Ann all night to just watch her. Make sure she was okay. So we made up a schedule for the kids to take shifts. Everyone wanted the first shift, none wanted the last. Connie finally got the first shift and the rest of us went to bed. Five minutes later Connie came in and said she couldn't do it. She was tired and Ann was crying. So I took the first shift. Ann and I sat in the rocking chair in the middle of the night with nobody around, getting to know each other.

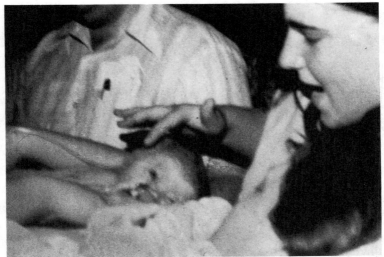

First Touch

Photo by Bobby

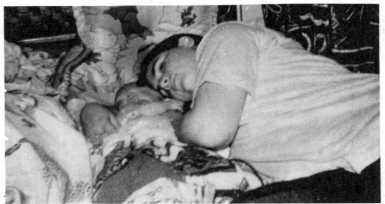

Photo by Bobby

Darling Ann

She was tired and needed to sleep. So after we looked at each other for a while and talked, (I talked with my mouth, she talked with her eyes.) and when she felt safe with me, she drifted asleep. Now I was exhausted, three days without sleep, but it didn't matter. Ann was more important so I took the second shift, too, and the third and the fourth. Finally I took her to Mom to nurse and left her in bed with Mom while I watched both of them. I wondered what any of us had done to deserve such an angel to give us such joy! It ended up that I watched her all night while everyone else slept. I wouldn't let the other kids get away with that for anyone but Ann.

146

SUSAN'S SONG TO ANN

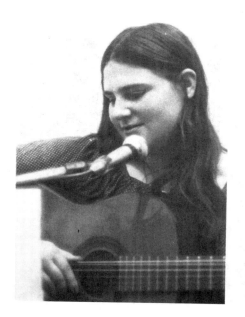

Written by Susan, Ann's first night with us.

Welcome to the world you pretty little girl
Welcome to the start of your life
Wishing on a star never got me far
until I saw the stars in your eyes could brighten up the skies

Your eyes make darkness sunshine
Your smile chases clouds away
And though you someday may wander
Your memory will always stay

Darling Ann, I love you when your near
And when you're gone I love you more
I know the way that you
looked in my eyes within minutes
of when you were born
Was the beginning of a friendship
That will last through all of our lives
I'm proud that you're my sister
And I'm glad that you're alive.

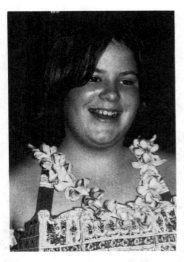

CONNIE'S STORY

(Age 13)

When Ann was born she was the ugliest glob of smelly stuff you have ever seen but after 36 hours of labor she was alive and that was all that mattered.

My mother miscarried the pregnancy before this one and they were so close that it seemed that she was pregnant continuously. (Living with a pregnant person

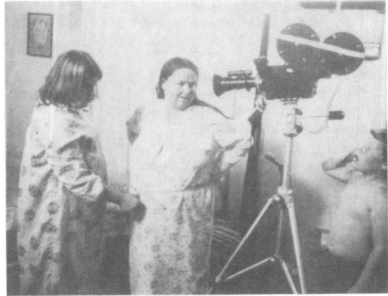

Photo by Gloria Goold

Connie measures, Bobby "directs"

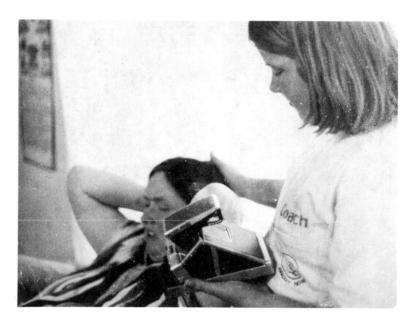

Connie the "Coach"

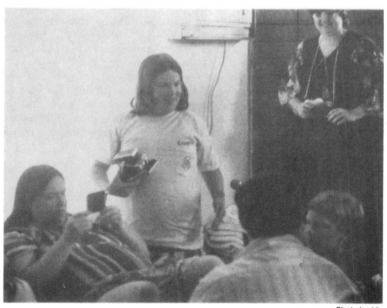

Connie takes pictures.

149

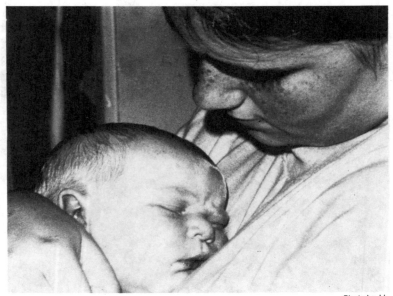

I'm glad that you're alive

for 18 months is not the easiest thing to do.) After the birth everyone was so excited that no one realized they were tired. On the way home it struck. It was hard to keep our eyes open. That night we all took shifts watching Ann, though I was too tired to do that, so I just knocked out. The next morning was Sunday and some of the family went to church but I was still sleeping.

On Monday I went to school loaded with pictures and stories. Not everyone was interested but some were. One of the teachers was going to send me to the office for bringing "those kind of pictures." It was only a picture of Ann nursing.

I think that children should be at the birth if they want to, but don't play favorites. If you have the eldest make the phone calls see that the younger one gets to make a few also. Make them feel important too.

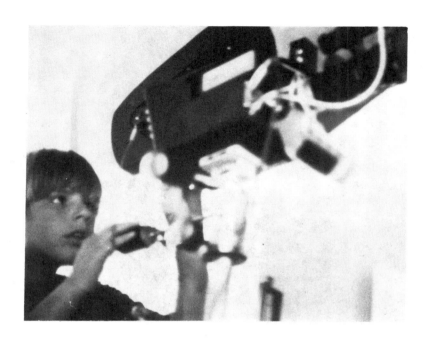

JJ'S STORY

(Age 11)

The first birth I was ever at was at this lady's house, but I don't remember that birth too well. Well, let's get on to another birth.

This one was at Dr. Berman's birth center. It all started when we got a call from Dr. Berman. He said if you want to film this birth. "You better get down here." So we got in our car and drove to the birth center. When we got there nothing was happening so we went and got some dinner.

When we got back, still nothing was happening, so we went to sleep there. At six in the morning she had her baby (see Jason Hatchell). It is really neat to watch a birth. It is a real miracle!

Ann's birth all started when Mom was carrying Erving. In early pregnancy my Mom was bleeding. The baby died when we were in Hawaii. I was going on a trip to Clear Creek on the day my Mom miscarried. I didn't find out until I got back. It was a terrible shock!

Two months later Mom was pregnant again. When she was in Chicago she started to bleed again, so we got worried about it, but it was all right.

Almost ten months went by. On October 7, 1977 she started to have the baby. The story started at 12:45 when my sister called. She wanted to know if anything was happening. Mom said everything is fine, but it wasn't. Then we

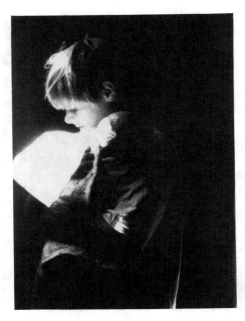

JJ - Brother

started getting ready. Then our sink got clogged-up and we had to fix the plumbing. After a long day we went to sleep. At two o'clock Mom woke Dad, and then woke us up. At four the Bermans came over, and so did everyone else. At eight we had breakfast.

That day we watched ton's of video-tapes. Finally at six we left for the birth center. We got my Mom in bed and she started pushing. Then all of a sudden Ann came out at 7:55.

None of the births I have been at have been scarey. It's amazing to watch a birth. Most people think its scarey and frightening, but it isn't. It's great to watch a birth! Still some people think it's terrible. Most people think it's terrible because they had knock-em-out drag-em-out obstetrics. That isn't natural childbirth.

Natural childbirth doesn't hurt as long as you move with the contraction and do not fight it.

It's really amazing how many mothers tell their children it's terrible and they don't want to talk about it..............

THE KINSELLAS
Bob's Views

There is a child present at every birth. When Marjie and Jay Hathaway asked me about our family decision to have our children present at our home birth, I realized that their presence had always been presumed, rather than decided.

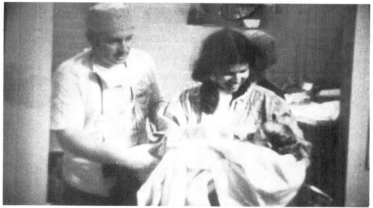

From the film "Childbirth for the Joy of It...Part II"

The Kinsellas and Erin - Their Seventh Birth

Upon reflection, their presence was a natural outgrowth of Jean's and my basic attitude that the children not only are a part of the family, but **are** the family.

I will never forget the comment made to me as a young teacher by my school principal when our first child, Lianne, was born, "Bob, now your life has really started." When Jean became pregnant with Denise, our second child, I remember how we spoke of the impact upon Lianne and how to involve her. When Roger came along, the girls were again involved.

I remember Renee's birth especially, because it was the first birth I had ever witnessed. I carried my excitment and enthusiam home to the three older children. There was special magic for them because "Dad" took them to the nursery school and picked them up. It was a fun and exciting time for everyone. Shawn's arrival is still clear in my mind because it was our first birth by the Bradley Method and the first time Jean came home from the hospital the same

153

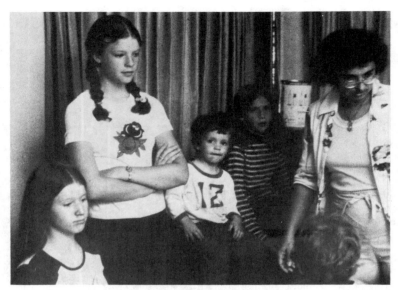

Lianne, Denise, Erin, Renee

day. The three older children came out to the car (the fourth was taking a nap) to greet Mom and Dad and their new little brother. Pictures of them at the car and later holding their new brother are family treasures.

When Ryan came along it was possible to video-tape his birth. This tape was later made into a film, which all of the children at home could enjoy. At some point we started having a birthday party with a big cake whenever we brought a new baby home. All of the children were able to enjoy a party and to celebrate the new arrival. Erin became the first child of ours to have his birth filmed and later used in the Bradley Method film, **Childbirth for the Joy of It - Part II**. All of our children have seen this film and many more.

Jean and I teach Bradley classes as a team, so childbirth is truly a natural part of our family environment. With Jean's eighth pregnancy it was decided to have a home birth. Our odyssey to this decision might well fill a separate book. We were interested in a natural birth, followed by a natural bonding, with a natural integration of the new member into the family unit.

As the time neared for Brendan's birth, no thought was ever given to not having the other children present. Jean and I spent our efforts in showing the kids films, discussing what to expect, and generally including them in all that you do to prepare for a new baby.

When Brendan did arrive, all of the children shared the moment of absolute excitement that I had first experienced with Renee's birth. We needed no long discussion of what happened because everyone had experienced what had happened.

Very recently it was emphasized to me just how involved and enthusiastic the other children were about being present at Brendan's birth. Jean is now pregnant with our ninth child. We have not said too much about our plans for the baby's

154

birth yet; that event still being a few months away. However, the other day several of the children came and asked if we planned to have the baby in a hospital or at home. When we replied that, of course, it would be at home, all of the kids present became excited and let out some "hurrays" because they would get to see the birth. If one child at a birth can bring so much happiness to the parents, consider how much more joy can be multiplied by other children present.

I believe that if parents will accept the fact that they are parents, having children present at everything will seem to be the natural way the family works. Almost every child has learned through TV how people are shot, stabbed, drowned, or strangled to death. I would hope that all children could have the experience of how someone is born to life as a counter-balance. All children have been present at their own birth. Why would anyone want to prevent them from sharing in someone else's birth?

Jean's Views

When I first sat down to write about "having our children present at our home birth", it seemed like a very difficult task. It was not possible to describe how we arrived at this momentous decision since a "decision" as such was never really made. Instead, it seemed normal and natural that our other children, numbering seven at the time would be included in such an important family event as the arrival of a new member.

It did occur to us that some of the children might have misgivings about being present at the birth. Therefore, we decided to let each child make his or her

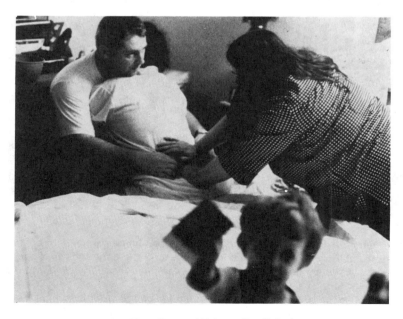

The Kinsellas and Erin — Marjie helps.

155

own decision. We called the children together and announced our decision to give birth at home. There was immediate excitement among the children.

Then we asked them how they would feel about being present. The general consensus was that it sounded like a neat idea but since none of the children had ever been present at a birth before, they wanted some time to think it over.

The answers were not long in coming. It was a unanimous, "Yes!"

My contractions began the night before the actual birth and continued through the following morning and afternoon. When the children awoke in the morning, no one wanted to go to school. After waiting for what seemed to them like "forever", each was afraid of missing out on the big event. I reassured them that the contractions were very mild, indicating that nothing much was happening. After promising to pick the children up from school should labor get active before the afternoon, they reluctantly left for school.

The little ones were, of course, home all day. They paid little attention to Mom who was home as usual. Instead they concentrated their energies on Dad who took a rare day off from work.

True to our prediction, labor got active shortly before the close of school that day. By the time the older children arrived home and the younger ones woke up

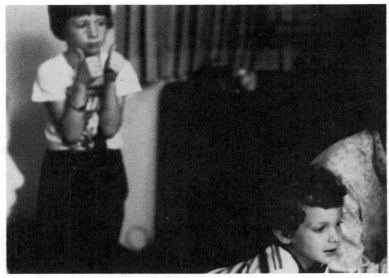

Shawn and Ryan

from their naps I was working hard with the contractions and was needing Bob's help to remain in control. Deep concentration on the contractions rendered me pretty much non-communicative other than an occasional "Hi" or a brief hug for the two-year-old.

The children seemed to sense our need for concentration and responded by quietly observing and from time to time drifting in or out of the room and helping out where needed. The two-year-old helped by rubbing "Mommy's" back.

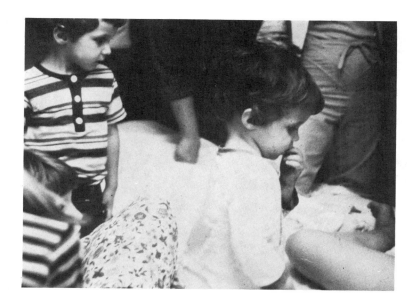

.Just when I decided that I was going to be in transition forever, I got the urge to push. Suddenly, all of the children appeared at the foot of the bed like a silent cheering section. The combined emotional support I received from Bob, who was supporting my shoulders and coaching me and from the children was really fantastic.

Physically, this was the most uncomfortable birth I had ever had since the baby was 9 lbs. 4 oz. and posterior; but emotionally it was the most relaxing of them all. I attribute that to being at home where Bob and I could share our birth with our children.

The sentiments of the children after the birth were, I believe, best summed up by the four-year-old. He came up to me the next day and said how neat he thought the birth had been and wanted to know if we could do that again tomorrow!

Lianne's Views
(Age 15)

When my Mom decided to have a home birth I became very excited. Imagine having a brother or sister at home! Of course, I had seen movies of a few of my brothers' births and other natural childbirth films, mainly Bradley, but it's nothing like really being there. I expected this birth to be fun and exciting. It was! But, it was a whole lot more.

When Mom started getting contractions it was the third day of school and so I decided to go, figuring that she would still be in labor by the time I got home. When I got home, sure enough she was still in labor. I was calm, but why shouldn't I be, I had only gone through this at least four times before. I went to the bedroom

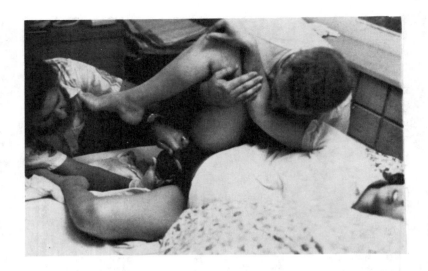

to see how things were going and after watching for a while, left very uncomfortable and a little scared. I am not used to seeimg my Mom in a lot of pain and discomfort. I came back only 10 to 15 minutes before the baby was born. The actual birth was interesting, but scarey.

The baby was an interesting purple color, but since it wasn't blue, I wasn't worried. The umbilical cord was a beautiful turquoise blue and the baby was very quiet. After Brendan was born I felt none of the "joy" one is supposed to feel when a baby is born — only relief that everything was all right. Then I held him and once again marveled at the newborn's tininess. It was after an hour that I began to feel that classic felling of joy of having a new addition to the family.

So, in the long run, it was a pleasurable experience and I am happy my parents let me (and the family) participate in the birth. Thanks.

Denise's Views
(Age 13)

I was at the birth of my little brother, Brendan, and I thought it was beautiful.

During the birth, nothing really frightened me because my parents had prepared us. I think it's important for anyone watching a birth to be prepared and to understand that having a baby is a lot of hard work.

I think it was important to be at Brendan's birth because now I can understand more fully what happens when a baby is born. I think I'm closer to Bren than if he had been born somewhere without the family being present.

Nothing was a shock to me but I was happy and surprised when, right after he was born, Bren hardly cried! I have a feeling that **he** was happier being born at home than the others who were born in the hospital. I may be remembering wrong, but Brendan seemed to have smiled and laughed right away, much sooner than the older children did.

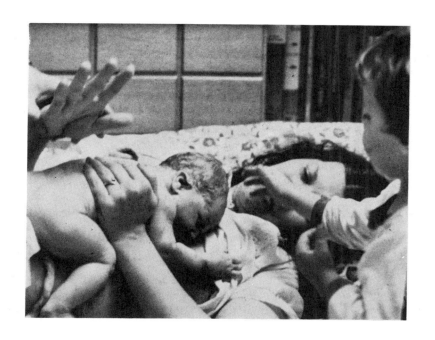

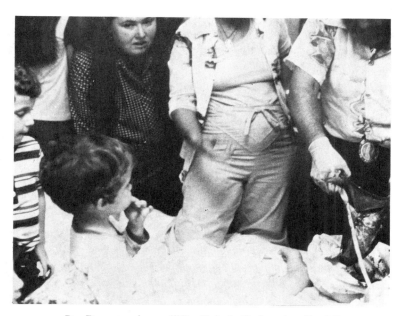

Dr. Berman shows "The Baby's Swimming Pool."

I was more excited and elated being present at the birth than I would have been if the baby had been born at the hospital. I was able to think about what had happened. It made me want to have children and, when I do, I plan to have my children at home with the family present.

The birthday of my baby brother was an experience I will never forget. It was one of the most beautiful and precious times of my life — something I want to save, to share with Bren when he gets older.

Roger's Views
(Age 11)

I was really excited about Mom having our baby at home. The way I see it, the baby was a present to the family from Mom and Dad. At first, we were all very excited. We gathered around the bed, watching, talking to Mom and Dad and each other.

Then, we wondered if Mom would have the baby that day or not. The little kids watched TV, Lianne and Denise sat in their room and talked, listened to the radio and did homework. I rode my bike.

As I rode around, I met a friend. We started talking and I told him my Mom was having a baby at home. He asked if I was excited and if so, why I wasn't there. I said that I was excited but nothing was going on. Just then Dad called me. I said "goodbye" real quick and left.

When I got home, the doctor had arrived and my Dad and he were helping Mom. She pushed with each contraction and we all were relieved when she stopped. Then, during the next contraction, the top of the baby's head appeared. Soon the entire head was there. We were all cheering her on and I prayed it would be a boy. Soon, after an awful lot of coaching and pushing, my prayers were answered. It was really wonderful to be there and I think if you know what's going on, it's a truly joyful experience.

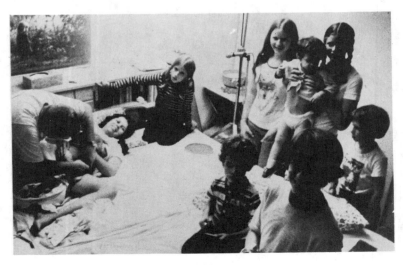

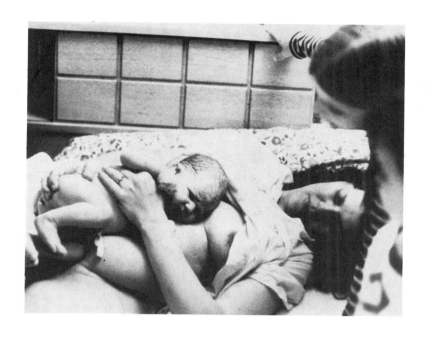

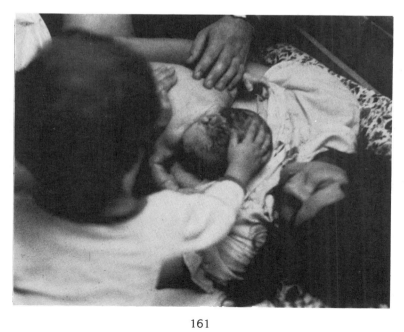

THE WINES' BIRTHS

By CHERYL & JERRY WINES, AAHCC

When we were expecting our third baby, a couple of friends had their children present at their home births. We couldn't see any reason not to and were comfortable with the idea. The excitement came when we told others of our plans. The reactions ranged everywhere from silent disbelief to outrage. It was inferred we were at best thoughtless and irresponsible parents. Predictably the strongest reactions came from the people in the generations who felt children should be "seen and not heard" and felt that sex was "not nice." Unfortunately, of course, both sets of Grandparents were included in this group.

In spite of our lack of support and certainly lacking any means of researching

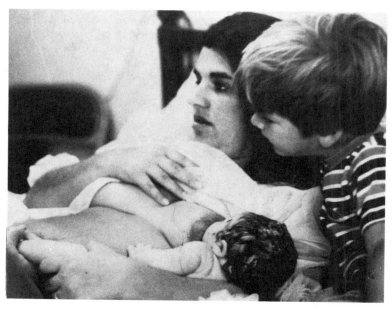

Jeff at Troy's Birth

163

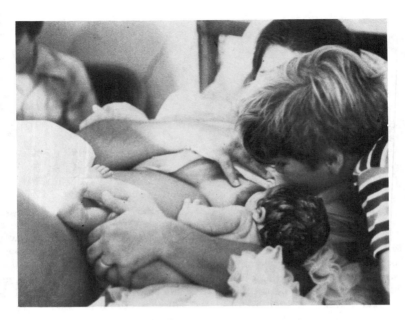

Jeff at Troy's Birth

this from experienced people, studies, or anything else, we had a sense that this was right for our children and ourselves. As it worked out, the delight in having our boys there was far beyond our expectations. They were amazingly sensitive, quiet, empathetic. They took their jobs (bringing ice chips, orange juice, wash rags, and so on.) very seriously, and the sweet, grinning faces when I looked up after the birth were priceless. Their comments and after-affects have never been anything but positive. But here — let's hear from the real experts:

"THE EXPERTS"

The first birth our sons, Jerry and Jeff, attended was when they were four-and-one-half and six-and-one-half years old. It was their brother Troy. Two years later they saw their third brother born, along with two-year-old Troy. When they were seven and nine, they were at the birth of a good friend. They are now nine and 11 and in a few months will again celebrate the birth-day of a new sibling. When I asked them whether they wanted to be at the birth, they all answered an emphatic "yes!". I asked each "Why?" The older boys looked at me quizzically and answered, "It's our baby!" Jeff said, "I want to see if it's a boy or a girl!" (I thought he still had a lot of optimism, considering). But, leave it to a four-year-old to sum it up. He said "It's going to be my birthday soon." I said, "Yes." Thinking we had lost our subject of conversation. "Will you and Dad and Jerry and Jeff and Todd come to my birthday?" I reassured him, "Of course, we would." "Well," he said, "It's going to be my baby's birth-day." Maybe that's the biggest difference in my children's attitudes. To them, this is all of our baby. Almost always when they talk, they refer to it as "our" baby or sometimes just "their" baby. They felt they had a **right** to be at the birth. I guess when you think about it, a baby is only made up of the mother and part of the father, but the same parts make up siblings, so in a way they are probably the closest possible relatives.

I loved their answers when I asked what children should know before they were at a birth. Naturally, I was anticipating that they would mention the blood, the water, and so on. All three answered exactly the same: "Make sure they know to be quiet!" They certainly had that lesson down. My oldest son added, "And the lights aren't too bright."

I must say their casual attitude bothered me at first. But then I started getting tickled at the look on their faces everytime I asked a question. I asked if anything ever was scarey at a birth. Again I get that strange look and "No! Like what??" I asked if Todd should be at this birth since he is so little (two years). They said, "It's his baby, too!!" Four-year-old Troy added, "Don't worry, he'll be bigger enough then." Nine-year-old Jeff said, "I'll be there to help him and take care of him if he needs anything." More and more it became apparent that my children feel birth is a normal, natural thing that happens — and most definitely a "family affair".

I asked the boys what they remembered most about Todd's birth. Jerry Paul

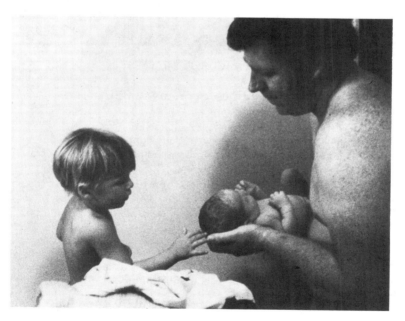

Troy and Daddy at Todd's Birth

said he liked seeing Dad "catch the baby." "It was fun." Jeff said he was happy when he got to hold Todd for the first time (about an hour after his birth). Troy said he gets a present from the baby and we have cake and ice cream. (Oh well, what can you expect, he was two years old when Todd was born).

165

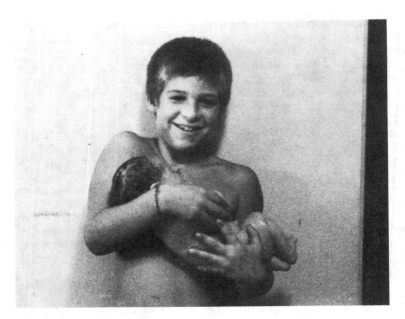

Jerry at Todd's Birth

Favorite Kid Quotes From Our Births

1973 - Troy's birth:
Dr. M.: "Why didn't you blow until I got here?"
4½-year-old Jeff: "Mom did!!" "Who blew the baby right out."
6½-year-old Jerry: "Can I take the cord for show-and-tell at school tomorrow?"

1975 - Todd's birth
9-year-old Jerry (next day): "Mom, would you come to school and tell my teacher I really was at the birth."
Jeff (7-years-old)(next day):
Mom: "Jeff, did you tell your class you were at the birth?"
Jeff: "I started to."
Mom: "What happened."
Jeff: "When I said I was at the birth, some of the kids asked me where the baby came from and a few of the other kids started laughing. I felt bad and didn't say anthing else. What was funny, Mom?"

Just recently (After a T.V. picture of a newborn baby in a hospital being spanked):11-year-Jerry Paul: "Mom, why did you have **me** in the **hospital** where they are mean to babies?"
Mom: "Parents have to learn and sometimes make mistakes. We didn't know how newborn babies should be treated until we learned after you were born."

MONICA'S BIRTH

Esperanza and George Quiroga were the first couple to have children at their birth at Sierra Madre Community Hospital in Southern California. Dr. Hai Abdul was her doctor.

What a marvelous opportunity to share our beautiful experience, even though we had it stored in our heart. Now writing it down will reinforce the value of those precious moments for the rest of our lives.

My due date was February 28. My husband and I had attended the Bradley Childbirth classes. We had done some reading on home birth and the security that it brings to the whole family. We wanted to be together and share every single moment at the miracle of birth, but because of some circumstances, we chose a hospital delivery. We worried about our three-year-old daughter, Diana, being left out, because we had seen some hospitals have a negative attitude toward parents' feelings. Thank God we chose the perfect doctor and the right hospital.

Diana was fully aware of her sister's expected birth. One of the reasons why she was so prepared was the fact that she was with us at the Bradley Classes from the very beginning.

It was February 25, at four in the morning, when we got to wrap Diana in a blanket while she slept still. We had arranged that my mom and sister would come with us, so my mother could hold Diana and my sister could take some pictures for all of us. Of course, with our doctor's approval. We finally got to the hospital at five in the morning. I was in such a hurry that I walked into the labor room while my husband, George parked the car. George met me at the labor room and started timing the contractions. We heard a discussion in the lobby and recognized the nurse's voice, not approving of our child being in the hospital. I was then 4 cm. dilated, so the nurse asked my husband to go back home and put Diana to bed. She felt I was going to have a long labor, and our daughter would be much better at home. I was shocked! I felt our dream of being all three in one at our baby's birth was going to be destroyed. I also felt our baby coming "any minute" and told George not to pay any attention and hold my hand. The nurse kept disapproving of the whole idea. After a couple of minutes our doctor came in and told us there was a misunderstanding on the nurse's part — she wasn't aware of the new hospital policy. We smiled and worked harder. At 6 a.m. I was ready to push so my family came into the labor room and shared and enjoyed our baby's waking up to life.

It was such a delightful experience seeing Diana smiling at her sister from the

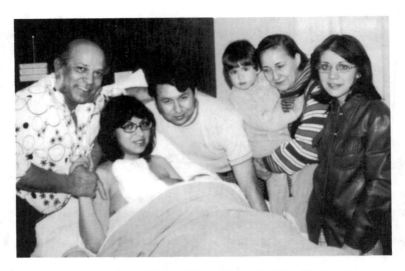

Monica nurses while Dr. Abdul congratulates the family.

first moment and holding her hand. I didn't feel the loneliness of knowing that she was home waiting for Mommy to come back. Instead we shared orange juice and hugged each other and came home together four hours after Monica was born.

I really thank God for putting in our way our doctor, our sweet Bradley teacher, and hope that every family can experience the same that we did, even at the hospitals.

LIVEA PRUE'S BIRTH

I was pleased to have my baby in a birth center for many reasons. But one that was very important to both myself and my husband, Marty, was being able to have our two-year-old daughter Ivy, present and part of the entire experience. I felt

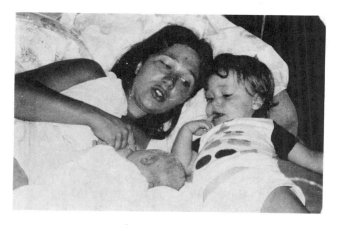

Sue, Livea and Ivy

certain that by including her in our birth she would be closer to and accept the the new little human with little or no difficulty.

I had a rapid-paced labor. I recognized what was transpiring at about 11 p.m. My husband made a bed for me with cushions and pillows on the floor in the back of our Volkswagen bus. His mother drove, with Ivy sleeping on the seat at her side. We live in Palmdale, about 65 miles away from the Nachis Birth Center in Culver City. We arrived at our destination around 1:30 a.m. Dr. Victor Berman and his wife Salee (also his nurse) met us at the rear door. I was examined. "We've got it made, nine centimeters," Vic said as his face lit up.

This was my second vaginal birth after a primary Cesarean section, and we were hoping for a rapid, uneventful labor. After pushing for about 20 minutes, the baby's head crowned and at that moment, my two-year-old, in the arms of my mother-in-law, rejoined us. As Livea was born, at 2:22 a.m., a friend that was

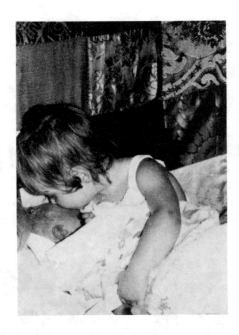

filming the birth for us, panned the camera to Ivy who looked on with wonderment on her face. As Marty and I were stroking and getting to know Livea, Ivy repeatedly talked about "her baby sister." She did not touch her until she was dressed, however. Dr. Berman had predicted that she wouldn't as he had observed several children her age at the birth of a sibbling and they've all followed the same pattern.

After Marty dressed the baby, Ivy climbed up on the bed and kissed her on the forehead. She hasn't stopped touching and loving her since and I can't help but think that my reason for wanting her to be present and a part of our birth was validated.

"I Helped Born Our Baby!"

By The Goold Family

"What kind of a parent would be so cruel as to subject a small child to the trauma of birth? It's impossible for them to comprehend what is happening, and it will undoubtedly leave them emotionally scarred for the rest of their lives."

This comment, made by a physician at a symposium on birth alternatives, was not a new refrain for me. I had heard the arguments again and again over the preceding year as people heard of our plan to include our three-year-old daughter in the birth of our new family addition. My response to the accusors was always the same, "Have you ever seen a child at a birth before? And, always the answer, "No! But, I have heard (or read) reports that show deep emotional trauma as a result of such an experience.

Baby Emily was four months old at the time of that particular confrontation.

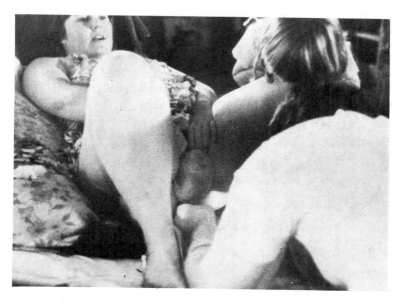

Jessica Watching Birth "I couldn't hardly believe my eyes!"

171

Our then almost four-year-old, Jessica was yet to show any signs of "trauma". In fact the excitement of the "Birth Day" was still so fresh in her memory that I was constantly on guard for unexpected references to it in public. Like the time we were in the check-out line at the supermarket and a lady behind us casually asked Jessica how she liked being a big sister. "It's real nice. I helped born baby Emily!" "I beg your pardon?" responded the lady. "I helped born our baby, and I cut the 'billical cord, and we had a party, and we planted the placenta under a tree for Emily, and . . ." I don't know what additional piece of information Jessica was about to share because the lady, (with a look of horror), had backed out of line mumbling something about needing some salt. Now, at almost six, and a full two years following Emily's Birth, Jessica is still full of enthusiastic memories of the "Birth Day." She has, however, come to understand that the choices we made for her little sister's birth are considered unusual to most people, and that it is a family subject that we don't share with just anyone.

Why did we choose to have Jessica participate in the birth? There are more reasons than I could even begin to list here. Some of the reasons stem from my own childhood where I can still vivdly recall the introduction of my "baby brother" into the family. Days of separation from my mother followed by a crying baby that I was constantly admonished "not to touch or get to close to." I can still recall how deeply I disliked that little intruder and how very many years it took he and I to develop a satisfactory relationship. I wanted Jessica's introduction to her sibling to be free from **that kind of trauma.** I also wanted her to have the opportunity to learn of nature's mysteries in a warm and loving way. This was a chance for her to learn first hand about the miracle of birth. Of all the reasons we decided to have

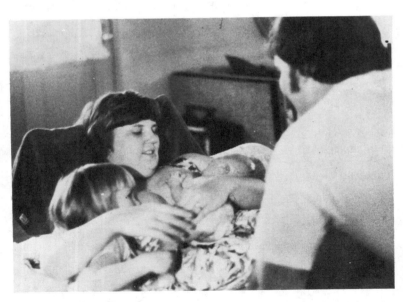

Breastfeeding Emily and Jessica — "Nummies for Baby Emily and me too!"

172

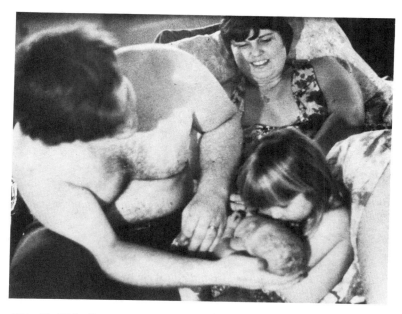

Skin-To-Skin Contact For Bonding. "I helped born you and I'm your big sister."

Jessica present, by far the most important, was the fact that she herself wanted very much to be there. We took great pains to prepare her for the experience and felt certain that there would be no surprises for her. She simply reflected our own attitude that this event was a good and natural thing.

How does Jessica remember her baby sister's "Birth Day"? Vividly I assure you, and with the unemcumbered innocence that is so typical of a child. When Emily was two months old I recorded the story of her birth just as Jessica related it to me from her own memory. She scrawled a set of pictures to illustrate "Her Story" and I think the reflections of Birth as she recorded them in their simplicity couldn't be more beautiful:

Emily's Story
By JESSICA LYNN GOOLD

First Mommy was pregnant and Emily was living in Mommy's uterus.

Mommy and Daddy and Me smile cause we love the baby.

Then one day labor started . . . and Jeff, and Jerry Paul, and Troy, and Todd, and Mrs. Wines and their Daddy came to help Mommy and Daddy born Emily.

We made the bed very beautiful and put everything on it and got ready. Then we waited, and waited, and waited, and waited, and waited.

Then all of a sudden Mommy pushed and pushed and Emily popped out, and cried a little bit. I couldn't hardly believe my eyes!

Then Mommy picked her up and nursed Emily . . . and me too!

I felt nice that the baby was here at last.

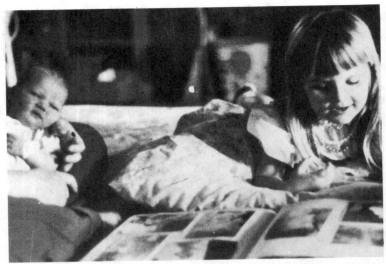

Showing "Daddy Pictures" from her own birth to her baby sister.

Then the placenta came right out and blood popped everywhere.
It got on everybody and me too.
But not on Ginger (our dog). The blood didn't hurt me.
The placenta felt soft like Emily.
We got out of bed and had a party.
We had cake and Emily gave me a highchair for my dollies.
Then Troy and everybody had to go.
Then we talked and looked at Emily and Mommy gave her more "nummies."
We were a family and felt very, very, very nice and happy that baby Em had been born.
The End.

Of course that wasn't the end, but only the beginning of a relationship between two sisters that began in a loving atmosphere and has grown and expanded beyond my wildest dreams. I am often asked if I think Jessica and Emily are closer because of the shared birth experience. Certainly I believe that that positive experience laid the foundation upon which a positive relationship could be built. How great an influence it has really had I can only speculate. I do know that the memory of that special Birth Day is a shared joy that each of us holds dearly in our hearts. I can think of no better way to bond a family together, each member in his special place, than through the shared miracle of Birth.

What kind of a parent would have his child present at Birth? I think perhaps it is that parent who truly understands the beauty and joy of that precious event, and is eager that his own children have the opportunity to witness and participate in one of life's truly miracles. The result . . . trauma? I think not! Rather an innocent acceptance of life's ever expanding circle. As a family we welcomed our newest edition into our arms. As for Jessica — her words say it best, "I helped born **OUR baby**".

REASONS BABIES
GIVE FOR NURSING

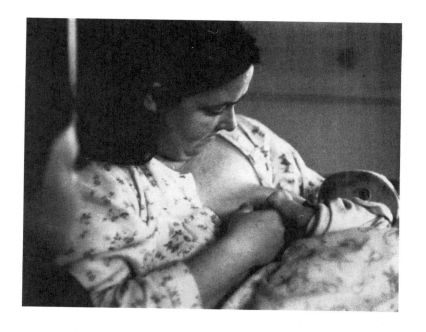

I'm hungry
I'm scared
I'm cold
I'm hurt
I'm bored
I love you

SPECIAL 'THANK YOU's

We would like to express our appreciation to the following people, without who's help, this book would not have happened:

The founding mothers of La Leche League, for inspiring us to trust in Nature, and for introducing us to Karen Osterlund, who introduced us to Dr. Robert Bradley, without his book *Husband-Coached Childbirth* birth would still be in the dark ages. Doris Haire, who opened our eyes, again, to the rightness of Natural Childbirth. Dr. Tom Brewer, who showed us the importance of eating right and said 'salt your food to taste'...like nature intended. To Vic and Salee Berman whose birth center encourages children at births. To the Kinsella family, whose births may someday fill a feature motion picture. To the Stewart Family, who show the way...by their example.

A special thank you to all who shared their own, personal messages in this book. To Cheryl Wines and Gloria Goold for their inspiration and encouragement, Pat Laubach, and Jalelah Fraley...for their examples. To Steve and Lisa Cushing for their support. To our own children for their love, understanding, and leadership. For Susan who said "it's about time that children had equal time!"

Thanks also to Elsie Gildersleeve and Bill Caldwell, for their professional expertise, and for working nights, and weekends to get this book out. A special 'thank's and 'sorry' to those we have forgotten to mention!

And to our parents, without whom we would not be here. WE LOVE YOU ALL!

177

BIRTHING AS A FAMILY IS REVOLUTIONARY !

Children at birth is a first of it's kind. It takes a previously forbidden topic and presents a positive, actually an emotional, case for having children present at siblings' births. The Hathaways explore the pros and cons, ending with an excitingly positive case for having siblings (who are well prepared) at birth. The "professional" interviews add authenticity but the chapter on the "Experts" viewpoint is the best. Children themselves report on how they felt seeing their brother or sister being born. The Hathaway children's stories are candid, interesting and thought provoking. Susan's Song to Ann is very emotional.

The section on choices is perhaps the most comprehensive up-to-date information available. Parents are really the ones responsible for their birth and their baby, and this chapter raises thought provoking issues that affect us all.

The Hathaways really make you think about all the "New" procedures that are being used, IV's, Fetal Monitors etc. Are they really better than the Natural process God intended ? ? ?

Perhaps the primary and most appealing aspect of the book is the over 125 pictures. How can anyone be a skeptic, after seeing so many births with children present? A picture is worth a thousand words.

<u>You</u> might ENJOY being a
CHILDBIRTH EDUCATOR!

* Teach a Method that WORKS!
* Give HONEST information!
* NATIONAL Affiliation!
* "800" HOT LINE for referrals!
* VIDEO available for classes!

A complete program. Academic requirements give background information. Personal workshop training from experts: in person, by film and video. Provisional teaching with personal attention. Enroll now to start training, and come to the workshop of your choice.

MISSOURI, Kansas City.....................October
CALIFORNIA, Los Angeles/ Disneyland .....No
WASHINGTON, DC / BALT.........November
FLORIDA, Fort Myers...........................March
HAWAII, Honolulu..................................Apr
TEXAS, Dallas...April
CALIFORNIA, Van Nuys..........................May
ILLINOIS, Chicago.................................May
NEW YORK, Orangeburg.........................June
CALIFORNIA, San Francisco....................July
WASHINGTON, Seattle...........................Augu
COLORADO, Denver............................August
GEORGIA, Atlanta.............................Septembe
NEW ENGLAND, Boston.......................Octobe
CALIFORNIA,Los Angeles/Disneyland.....Nov.
WASHINGTON DC, Manassas............Decembe
ARIZONA, Phoenix.........................December

The Bradley Method®
TOLL FREE (800) 423-2397
In California (818) 788-6662, or (800) 42-BIRTH
Approved by California Board of Registered Nursing (Provider 06211)

NOTE:

This is a typical year's schedule... Please call or write for specific dates and details of workshops in the future.